T'ai Chi Fundamentals

For Health Care Professionals and Instructors
A Simplified Approach for Mastering T'ai Chi Basics

Tricia Yu MA
Jill Johnson MS PT GCS

Uncharted Country Publishing
Madison, Wisconsin

D1264733

Uncharted Country Publishing
P.O. Box 756
Taos, New Mexico 87571

www.taichihealth.com
800-488-4940

Book design by Earl J. Madden
Cover design by Kai Yu
Photography by Jim Wildeman
Calligraphy by Robert Lin-I Yu
Printed by Litho Productions

Dedicated to our parents:

Robert and Mildred Beadles
Cleon and Irene Johnson

Thanks to T'ai Chi Masters Benjamin Pang Jeng Lo, William C.C. Chen and Liu Pei Ch'ung for your patience. Special thanks to the inspirational students in the T'ai Chi Fundamentals Class, to Lauri McKean for your work plans, muffins, creativity and laughter, to Sarah Carroll for your Virgo focus during time off from the circus trapeze, to Betty Chewning for your steadfast light, to Gabrielle Byers for your teaching spirit at the T'ai Chi Center, to Dianne Molvig for your editorial clarity, to Charles Meyers for your loving support, and to Doug Swayne for making all of this possible.

OVERVIEW
The T'ai Chi Fundamentals Program

T'ai Chi Fundamentals presents a simplified, systematic approach for mastering T'ai Chi basics. It is designed to make T'ai Chi accessible to most ambulatory adults while maintaining the integrity of traditional Yang Style form. The program includes the following three elements:

1. The Movement Patterns
These are are a series of exercises designed to reinforce important functional movements repeated throughout the T'ai Chi form. These take 4-11 minutes to perform, depending on the number of repetitions.

2. The Fundamentals Form
This is a simplified sequence of movements from traditional Yang Style T'ai Chi that takes less than 5 minutes to perform.

3. The Mind/Body Principles
These serve as guidelines for practicing the movements and enhance the experience of well-being.

The program is presented in three sections. The first section introduces simple functional movements and the later sections progress to movements that are more challenging.

Program Background

Tricia Yu developed **T'ai Chi Fundamentals** based on 28 years' experience teaching Yang Style T'ai Chi. She identified consistent areas of difficulty that students encountered in learning T'ai Chi and targeted critical elements from the traditional form that enhance balance, coordination, strength and endurance.

She has taught this program for three years to healthy older adults and to those with conditions ranging from arthritis, fibromyalgia and heart disease to gastrointestinal problems, cancer and orthopedic injuries. Two health maintenance organizations reimburse their subscribers for participation in this community-based wellness program.

Jill Johnson analyzed the Movement Patterns of the T'ai Chi Fundamentals Program for their clinical applications and functional benefits. She found that the specific Movement Patterns follow a motor development progression and can be used as tools for patient assessment and intervention. A practitioner of T'ai Chi herself, Jill uses elements of this program as a therapeutic intervention for her geriatric clientele.

Program Resources

This text is one part of a multimedia instructional resource designed to assist instructors in learning and teaching **T'ai Chi Fundamentals**. In addition, there are video and audio resources which are described in detail below:

Resources for Health Professionals and Instructors:

VIDEO: *T'ai Chi Fundamentals for Health Care Professionals and Instructors* includes the following:

- **Introduction** to the history, philosophy, health benefits and practical applications of T'ai Chi.
- **Demonstration** of the entire Fundamentals Form.
- **Instruction** in the Fundamentals Form, the Movement Patterns and Mind/Body Principles in three sections that progress in difficulty. Each section includes:
  - Analysis of the clinical applications and functional benefits of the movements.
  - Outline of basic T'ai Chi principles.
  - Instruction and guided practice for the Movement Patterns.
  - Instruction and guided practice for the Fundamentals Form.
  - Perspectives for integrating T'ai Chi practice into daily life.
- **Guided Practice** of all Movement Patterns.

TEXT: *T'ai Chi Fundamentals for Health Care Professionals and Instructors: A Simplified Approach for Mastering T'ai Chi Basics* is designed to be used in conjunction with the video. It expands the discussion on clinical and therapeutic applications and describes modifications from the traditional Yang Style Form. In addition, it includes further information and references useful both to health care professionals and experienced T'ai Chi practitioners.

AUDIO: *The T'ai Chi Fundamentals Form* provides detailed instruction for performing the movements of the Fundamentals Form. It is for both instructors and students.

Resources for Patients and Students:

VIDEO: *T'ai Chi Fundamentals: Simplified Exercises for Beginners* is designed as a resource to support daily home practice. It is an essential tool for patient and student learning. It includes the **Introduction, Principles, Instruction, Perspective and Guided Practice** portions from the above video.

AUDIO: (same as above).

Table of Contents

CHAPTER ONE
Elements of T'ai Chi Fundamentals

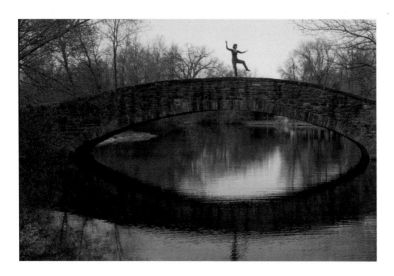

Introduction

T'ai Chi Ch'uan, (also written "Taiji" or "Taijiquan") is commonly referred to simply as "T'ai Chi." It is a slow, graceful Chinese exercise that enhances relaxation skills, mental focus and physical alignment while building leg strength, endurance and stability. Ideal for increasing stamina, flexibility and coordination, T'ai Chi promotes efficiency of movement and economy of effort. Its principles apply to all activity. T'ai Chi is a form of *Qigong*, a Chinese term for energy cultivation.

As medical research validates the benefits of T'ai Chi practice, health professionals are seeking training in this Chinese exercise in order to evaluate its applications as a complementary therapy. Growing numbers of older adults as well as those with pain and physical limitations are also exploring T'ai Chi as an alternative exercise. In addition, many community-based classes and wellness programs are including T'ai Chi in their curricula. Individuals of all ages and physical abilities are finding their way into T'ai Chi classes. However, this ancient exercise remains elusive to many who find its slow, complex movements confusing and difficult to master.

The T'ai Chi Fundamentals Program

Description

T'ai Chi Fundamentals bridges eastern mind/body health principles with western medical model functional analysis. The first program of its kind, it provides a simplified approach for mastering T'ai Chi basics and describes T'ai Chi in terms that are useful to health care professionals. It presents a clear, systematic sequence for learning the movements of T'ai Chi and introduces components of T'ai Chi practice that facilitate both mental and physical well-being. T'ai Chi Fundamentals can serve as a complete exercise program for many individuals. In addition, it can provide solid basic training for those who wish to progress to the more complex forms of traditional T'ai Chi.

The program includes three primary components:

1. It introduces the **Movement Patterns**. These are a series of exercises that are practiced to reinforce the body positions repeated throughout the T'ai Chi form.
2. It offers step-by-step instruction in the **Fundamentals Form.** This is a simplified version of T'ai Chi based in traditional movements.
3. Finally, this program introduces important **Mind/Body Principles** which serve as guidelines for T'ai Chi practice.

Rationale

Accessibility: T'ai Chi Fundamentals is designed to bring the many benefits of T'ai Chi to individuals with a wide range of abilities. It can be taught by health professionals to their clients, in classes for older adults and to those with limiting conditions. This program also can be a creative tool for T'ai Chi instructors who are teaching introductory courses. It may be useful in classes of all experience levels for reinforcing practice of basic postures and movements of T'ai Chi.

Standardization: The T'ai-Chi Fundamentals Program is designed systematically and can be used as a standard to facilitate research which can contribute to a greater understanding of the benefits and contraindications of this exercise. During the past 10 years, there has been a small body of research on T'ai Chi. Preliminary studies suggest that T'ai Chi practice may have positive physical and mental health outcomes. However, one impediment to widespread use of T'ai Chi for research or as a clinical health intervention has been the lack of one specific set of exercises or basic movement components that constitute a standard T'ai Chi form.

The term "T'ai Chi," encompasses several styles, each originating from three main branches named after their most famous proponents (Yang, Chen or Wu). To add to the confusion, many interpretations of these styles have emerged throughout its long history, resulting in numerous variations in form. All these traditional forms of T'ai-Chi involve highly complex movement patterns that take months or years to learn. In the past, controlled studies have involved a version of one of these styles that has been personally abbreviated by an instructor in order to provide the subjects with something they can learn in a few weeks. To address this issue, the T'ai-Chi Fundamentals Form provides a standard movement sequence that follows a systematic motor development progression. It is based in Yang Style T'ai Chi, the most widely practiced form worldwide. Designed with discrete, measurable increments in difficulty, it may have broad application for researching outcomes for individuals whose abilities range from limited function to advanced athletic skills.

Assessment and Treatment: The Movement Patterns in this program follow a motor development progression and can be used as tools for both client assessment and intervention. By observing performance of these movements, the teacher or therapist can assess misalignments which might contribute to physical limitations. These precise patterns then can be used in the client's exercise program or as treatment strategies. They also can be prescribed for daily practice to help correct these problem areas.

Precautions

This program is not intended as a substitute for medical consultation. Remind your patients and students to consult with a physician or therapist before embarking on this or any exercise program.

Some Comparisons Between Traditional T'ai Chi and T'ai Chi Fundamentals

Characteristics of Traditional T'ai Chi Forms

T'ai Chi was originally developed by Chinese martial arts experts in order to advance their skills. Traditional T'ai Chi forms incorporate highly complex movement patterns throughout the entire sequence which are based in blocks, kicks and punches. Most traditional forms take 12-20 minutes to perform and over one year to learn. Although natural athletic ability and previous movement training are a great asset, the discipline of regular practice is the key to long-term benefits. T'ai Chi, like any true art, has a depth which can be appreciated through years of practice and dedication. As many T'ai Chi students will affirm, it takes a lifetime to learn.

T'ai Chi incorporates principles for health of body, mind and spirit. These principles promote harmony in human interactions as well.

Characteristics of The T'ai Chi Fundamentals Program

This program offers a simplified, systematic approach for mastering T'ai Chi basics which maintains the integrity of traditional form and principles. It modifies or eliminates problem areas that students consistently encounter when learning T'ai Chi and provides essential groundwork for learning the traditional Yang Style Form. It includes the following three elements:

1. The T'ai Chi Fundamentals Form is an exercise form that adapts the movements and principles of traditional Yang Style T'ai Chi Ch'uan into a practice routine that is accessible to people with a wide range of abilities. In addition, it targets critical elements from the traditional form which enhance balance, coordination, strength and endurance. Each section can be practiced as a complete and challenging program depending on the abilities of the participant. It takes less than five minutes to perform.

The T'ai Chi Fundamentals Form is taught in three sections. It incorporates the most basic and essential functional movement components in the first section, and progresses to more complex patterns in the later sections. It eliminates some of the more difficult details of the traditional form that relate specifically to martial arts applications. This step-by step method provides an accessible approach for developing skills necessary for performing the entire sequence, and is a vehicle for clearly learning the movements.

2. The Movement Patterns are a series of twelve exercises designed to reinforce important functional movements repeated in the Fundamentals Form. In addition, these patterns integrate expressive arm movements and elements of *Qigong* energy cultivation into the exercises. Like the Fundamentals Form, the specific Movement Patterns follow a motor development progression. Each Movement Pattern is practiced repetitively as a vehicle for training T'ai Chi skills. They are also enjoyable, expressive, complete and challenging as an exercise program on their own. They take 4-12 minutes to perform, depending on the number of repetitions.

3. The Mind/Body Principles describe elements of T'ai Chi practice that enhance physical and emotional well-being. These principles are guidelines for healthy human interaction as well.

Summary: Characteristics of Traditional T'ai Chi

- Developed by Chinese martial arts experts in order to advance their skills.
- Incorporates highly complex movements throughout the entire sequence.
- Includes one set sequence of movements that takes 12-20 minutes to perform.
- Is learned most easily by individuals with some movement training.
- Includes mind/body principles that serve as guidelines for T'ai Chi practice.

Summary: Characteristics of T'ai Chi Fundamentals

- Developed as a simplified version of traditional Yang Style T'ai Chi with emphasis on balance, coordination, strength and endurance.
- Incorporates movements which progress in difficulty. The first section introduces simple functional movements, and the following two sections progress to movements that are more complex.
- Includes two sets of exercises:
  - The **Movement Patterns**: a series of exercises designed to reinforce important functional movements repeated throughout the T'ai Chi form. They take 4-11 minutes to perform, depending on the number of repetitions
  - The **Fundamentals Form**, a simplified T'ai Chi form that takes less than 5 minutes to perform.
- Is accessible to most ambulatory adults.
- Includes **Mind/Body Principles** that serve as guidelines for T'ai Chi practice.

Overview Of T'ai Chi

Origins

T'ai Chi originated in China around the 13th century A.D. as a synthesis of martial arts exercise and sitting meditation. The perspective of the *Tao* was intregal to the philosophy and culture of China for thousands of years and naturally influenced the development of T'ai Chi. *Tao* is translated as "road" or "path." The *Tao* is a path for living in harmony with the earth and with other humans. According to this perspective, living simply, being quiet and observant and willing to move with the flow of things promotes long and harmonious life. This insight is based on astute observation of nature's cycles and on a cosmology that is compatible with modern theoretical physics.

Ancient naturalists and astronomers spent time each day observing their own inner process and meditating on the rhythms and currents within their own bodies. They realized that the body is a microcosm of the universe and that one's personal health is influenced by the rhythmns of life on earth, the patterns of the larger universe, and all relationships to other humans. All of life is interconnected. Over time, this exploration of inner realms produced an intricate map of the energy conduits or acupuncture meridians within the body through which *Qi* or "life force" flows.

This process had an influence on the martial arts. T'ai Chi, which is based on self defense movements, evolved as a physical activity for integrating mind, body and spirit to function in harmony with the external world. Rather than cultivating brute force, which inevitably becomes depleted. T'ai Chi (which means "Supreme Ultimate") cultivates The Middle Way, a peaceful path.

Recent History

For many centuries, T'ai Chi was practiced privately, passed on from father to son in the Chen Village in northern China. Beginning in the mid-1800's Master Yang Lu Shan, founder of the Yang Style form, was the first to teach T'ai Chi publicly. It soon became popular in martial arts circles as an advanced self-defense method. In the early 20th century Lu Shan's grandson, Master Yang Cheng Fu promoted T'ai Chi as a health exercise. Since then, it has enjoyed widespread popularity in China. Adults of all ages practice the flowing postures every day. Many older adults begin learning Tai Chi after retirement.

Each morning, parks in China's large cities are filled with people performing this ancient exercise. Early risers do their round of T'ai Chi before going to work, while later arrivals include retired elderly who come to socialize as well as practice. Any day, in almost any weather, millions of people in China are practicing T'ai Chi.

T'ai Chi in the West

In the late sixties, T'ai Chi began to take root in the United States and Europe. Grand Master Cheng Man Ching, of the Yang Style lineage, came to New York and was one of the first to teach this ancient exercise openly to non-Chinese students. Since then, Masters Benjamin Pang Jeng Lo and William C.C. Chen and other Yang Style teachers have taught T'ai Chi to thousands of students across the United States and Europe, making it the most popular form worldwide. In addition to Yang Style, the Chen and Wu systems of T'ai Chi are growing in popularity. Increasing numbers of people are finding this combination of movement and mental focus an excellent approach to both physical fitness and stress reduction.

Health Benefits

Recent medical research has brought the many benefits of T'ai Chi to the attention of health professionals. T'ai Chi is a weight-bearing and moderate-intensity cardiovascular exercise. Current research suggests that practice of T'ai Chi can improve balance, reduce falls and increase leg strength. It also can lower blood pressure and stress hormones, enhance respiratory and immune function, and promote emotional well-being. (See Appendix: **Summary of Research.**)

Clinical Description

T'ai Chi facilitates postural reintegration and diaphragmatic breathing, and promotes physiological indicators of the Relaxation Response. In addition, it facilitates proper body mechanics and increased kinesthetic and proprioceptive awareness. It involves rotation of all major joints, but not to their full range. It is gentle exercise suitable for all ambulatory adults.

Perspective from a T'ai Chi Master

T'ai Chi Master William C. C. Chen outlines his objectives for T'ai Chi practice as follows:
• Simple
• Easy
• Natural
• Enjoyable
• Productive

Guidelines for T'ai Chi Practice

Mindfulness

Basic to the practice of T'ai Chi is an attitude of mindfulness, or awareness of the present moment. Attention is focused on the position and feeling within the body. Surroundings are experienced with the senses. In that T'ai Chi requires mental focus, it is critical that the practitioner take a moment to bring full attention to the present before beginning the sequence. During practice, the mind naturally wanders. The practitioner simply refocuses on the movements, or monitors balance, posture or breathing in order to redirect attention into the present moment.

Postural Alignment

The practitioner maintains focus on standing postural alignment throughout the sequence, checking to see that the body is upright, the head erect, spine comfortably aligned, shoulders balanced and relaxed, and the weight evenly distributed on the soles of the feet. While moving, the body remains in an upright position and the shoulders remain aligned over the hips.

Breath Awareness

Natural diaphragmatic breathing patterns are maintained throughout the entire sequence. Many people hold their breath while concentrating. T'ai Chi trains breath awareness with movement.

Active Relaxation

Many people are unaware of the tension they hold in their bodies. Active relaxation involves integrating mindfulness with physical relaxation and facilitates simultaneous awareness of all parts of the body. It involves being both alert and calm at the same time and promotes the flow of *Qi* or life force throughout the body. T'ai Chi training reinforces active relaxation, both when being still and when in motion. Like any skill, it is learned gradually through practice.

Slow Movement

Most exercise programs focus on exertion and straining as a means to achieving increased strength and endurance. T'ai Chi facilitates both strength and endurance through slow, relaxed movement. With the knees bent and the body relaxed in proper alignment, dramatic load-bearing benefits occur. The continuous movement in a flexed stance promotes endurance. The slower and lower the movement, the greater the strength and endurance benefit.

Weight Separation

During transitions and weight shifts onto the back foot, the weight ideally is 100 percent on one foot, keeping the body upright. Commonly referred to as "separating the weight," it contributes to better balance and increased leg strength.

Integrated Movement

The head, trunk and pelvis rotate as a single "column" aligned over the stable base in the feet. All arm and hand movements are initiated by the upright rotation of this "column." There is no twisting of the spine.

Guidelines from a T'ai Chi Master

T'ai Chi Master Benjamin Pang Jeng Lo summarizes guidelines for practice in his Five Basic Principles as follows:
- **Relax** (Mindfulness, Active Relaxation).
- **Body Upright** (Postural Alignment).
- **Separate Yin and Yang** (Weight Separation).
- **Move from the Waist** (Integrated Movement).
- **Keep Fair Lady's Wrist** (wrists neutral, element of Active Relaxation).

CHAPTER TWO
The Movement Patterns

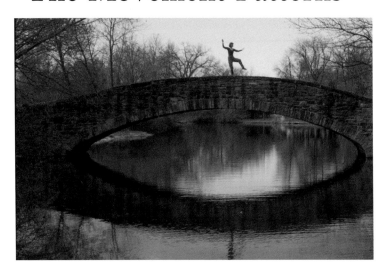

Description

This chapter includes **Reminders** for practice of each Movement Pattern, an outline of their physical and emotional **Benefits, Discussion** of functional applications, and **Quotes from the T'ai Chi Masters** regarding performance of these movements.

The Movement Patterns provide training in the essential skills of T'ai Chi and facilitate postural realignment, increased leg strength, balance, endurance and coordination. They are designed as warm-ups to the form and can stand alone as an enjoyable exercise program. Practice of these movements also can reinforce performance of specific movements of the T'ai Chi Fundamentals Form. Each pattern integrates the skills from the preceding movement and progresses in difficulty.

The Movement Patterns represent a synthesis of Eastern and Western, ancient and modern exercises. They include traditional T'ai Chi warm-up exercises, variations on ancient Bear and Crane Qigong, and creative, expressive movement.

Traditional T'ai Chi movements are based in martial arts blocks and punches. The arms are positioned in front of the body to protect the trunk. The Movement Patterns include open, expressive arm movements adding cardiovascular, range of motion and emotional benefits to the program.

Names of the Movement Patterns

Section One:
Posture and Breathing
Arm Swinging
Crane Takes Flight
Open and Stable
Bear Rooting
Bear Walk

Section Two:
Basic Bear
Holding the Moon
The Ski Move

Section Three:
Flying Crane
Softball Pitch
Dancing Crane

The Movement Patterns of Section One

The Movement Patterns of this section represent essential components of basic functional skills and can constitute a complete and challenging program. Many patients can achieve their rehabilitation goals by mastering Section One. It is recommended that patients progress to Section Two only when deemed appropriate by their health care provider.

In a classroom setting, the Movement Patterns can be practiced as part of a warm-up routine and can reinforce learning of specific patterns of functional movement which are repeated throughout the form.

"The upright body must be stable and comfortable."
Wu Yu-Hsiang

"When the coccyx is straight, the spirit goes through to the head top."
Unknown author, T'ai Chi Classics

"To make the whole body light and agile, suspend the head top."
Unknown author, T'ai Chi Classics

Posture

The basic T'ai Chi posture emphasizes relaxed, natural body alignment.

Movements

1. **Horse Stance, Center Position:** both feet are flat, parallel, hip-distance apart with knees slightly bent. Weight is evenly distributed between both feet.

Reminders

- "Head as if suspended from above" involves an uplift at the crown, called the *Bai Hui* or "Hundred Channels Point" in Chinese acupuncture. There is also an uplift at the occiput or "Jade Pillow."
- Eyes are relaxed with a level forward gaze that includes awareness of the periphery.
- Chin is relaxed so that the teeth are separate. Mouth is closed with the lips lightly touching.
- Shoulders are even and relaxed in standard alignment.
- Pelvis is relaxed in a neutral position. Tailbone is in line with the heels.
- Weight is evenly distributed over the entire sole of each foot.

Benefits

- Natural alignment reduces stress on the neck, shoulders and spine.
- Balance is enhanced when the knees are slightly bent and weight is evenly distributed over the feet.

Discussion

Awareness of body position is an important element of mind/body integration. Routinely checking into head, shoulder and spine position can facilitate increased subtle awareness within the body.

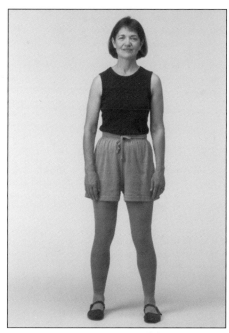

1. Horse Stance, Center Position

Breathing

T'ai Chi is practiced with a focus on diaphragmatic or natural belly breathing.

Movements

1. **Diaphragmatic Breathing:** breathe in, let the belly relax and expand. Then breathe out and it naturally contracts.

Reminders

- Feel the movement within the body when breathing. Relax.
- The belly feels as though it is filling up with the inhalation, and as if it is emptying with the exhalation.

Benefits:

- Natural deep-breathing patterns allow the lungs to fill completely with air, oxygenating every cell.
- Natural diaphragmatic breathing is the beginning step in cultivating an increased sense of vitality or vital energy, which the Chinese call *Qi* (also spelled *Ch'i*) .

Discussion

Shallow breathing patterns are characteristic of many adults in Western cultures. Chronically tensing the abdominal muscles in order to maintain a flat stomach reduces oxygen intake and can contribute to anxiety. In addition, inhibiting the natural expansion and contraction of the belly while breathing contributes to reduced muscle tone in the abdominal region. During natural belly breathing, there is continuous contraction and co-contraction of abdominal muscles, facilitating healthy muscle tone in that region.

People may benefit from simply focusing on feeling the movement in their body as they breathe. For many, it is easier to experience diaphragmatic breathing while lying down.

According to the T'ai Chi Classics, the body's storehouse of energy is located in the belly. Called the *Dan Tien* or "Cinnabar Field," this area is energized by combining natural diaphragmatic breathing with a relaxed focus on the breath. This helps bathe the inner organs with vital energy.

"T'ai Chi Ch'uan is based on the natural way of breathing: it is slow, gentle and deep."
William C.C. Chen

The abdomen relaxes and the breath sinks."
Wu Yu-Hsiang

"Completely relax the abdomen."
T'ai Chi Classics, unknown author

"The inhalation and exhalation are long and deep and the ch'i sinks to the Tan T'ien."
Yang Cheng Fu

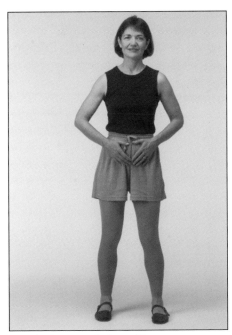

1. Diaphragmatic Breathing

Arm Swinging

The entire Tai Chi Form is done with relaxed arms. **Arm Swinging**, based in a Chinese *Qigong* exercise, helps facilitate this movement.

"Sink shoulders and elbows."
Yang Cheng Fu

"The shoulders will be completely relaxed and open."
Chen Wei Ming

Movements

1. **Horse Stance, Center Position:** swing arms slightly forward.
2. **Horse Stance, Center Position:** swing arms slightly backward.

Reminders

- **Horse Stance** (see **Posture,** page 14).
- Arms move like ropes or pendulums dangling from the shoulders.
- Keep the head and shoulders relaxed.
- If shoulders and elbows are relaxed, swing higher.

Benefits

- This exercise can help release tension in the neck and shoulders.
- Arm swinging contributes to increased synovial fluid to the shoulder joint.
- The movement may stimulate the lymph glands.

Discussion

Use **Arm Swinging** to encourage arm relaxation which is integral to the practice of T'ai Chi. This movement may be helpful for patients who have had shoulder surgery or for anyone who has arthritis or a frozen shoulder. It can also be of great benefit to individuals who have lost normal arm swing during gait. It can be the next progression from the standard Codman's exercise, which is done with gravity eliminated. By progressing to an upright position, **Arm Swinging** works more against gravity and helps loosen the shoulder.

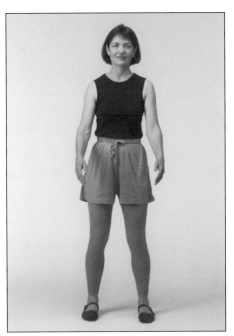

1. Horse Stance, Center Position;
arms swing forward

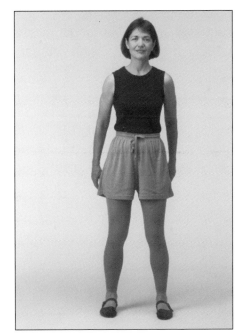

2. Horse Stance, Center Position;
arms swing back

Crane Takes Flight

This is based on ancient *Qigong* exercises inspired by animal movements. It provides practice for the T'ai Chi form which is done entirely with the knees bent.

"—you must first strengthen the two thighs and loosen the shoulders and let the qi sink down."
Li I Yu

"No leaning "
Benjamin Pang Jeng Lo

"In motion, all parts of the body must be light, nimble and strung together."
Chang San Feng

Movements

1. **Horse Stance, Center Position:** bend knees, lowering arms at sides.
2. **Horse Stance, Center Position:** straighten knees raising arms at sides.

Reminders

- Begin with the feet in the **Horse Stance, Center Position** (see **Posture**, page 14), feet pointing straight ahead, hip-distance apart.
- Weight remains evenly distributed over the soles of both feet.
- Knees stay in alignment with the feet throughout the movement.
- Tailbone stays in line with the heels.
- Pelvis remains in a neutral position.
- Trunk maintains an upright position.
- Arms stay relaxed while working against gravity.
- Shoulders stay relaxed throughout the movement.
- Elbows stay slightly bent through out the movement.
- Wrists are flexed as arms are raised, and extended as they lower.

Benefits

- This movement strengthens the quadriceps, minimizing stress to the knee joint.
- Ankle dorsiflexion, necessary for good balance, is often lacking in older adults. This movement promotes greater ankle range of motion. Increased ankle dorsiflexion allows more weight to transfer evenly onto the balls and heels of the feet.
- Keeping the back straight minimizes stress to the back.
- The arm movements are optional depending on a person's balance and coordination.
- Slow, relaxed movement reduces stress to the joints and improves kinesthetic and proprioceptive awareness.
- Arm movements add a cardiovascular benefit.
- This movement is important for transfers, such as getting in and out of the bathtub and for lifting.

Discussion

As the body is lowered, many people have trouble staying upright and keeping the pelvis in a neutral position. Therefore it may be beneficial to initially use support in order to maintain balance. Use this Movement Pattern for individuals with weak quadriceps and/or poor ankle range of motion. It is excellent preparation for transfer training.

This movement can be used to practice coordinating movement with breathing. Inhale as arms are raised, exhale as they are lowered.

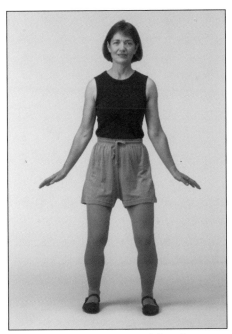

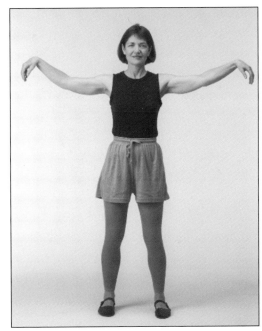

1. Horse Stance, Center Position, knees bent; arms lowered at sides

2. Horse Stance, Center Position, knees straightened; arms raised at sides

The Stable and Open Move

This pattern prepares for transition movements in T'ai Chi. One leg remains stable as the other rotates externally.

Movements

1. **Stable and Open Move:** arms open expressively as the knees bend and the weight shifts onto one leg. The other leg rotates externally.
2. **Horse Stance, Center Position:** arms in front of the body as if holding a large ball. Fingertips face each other at midline without touching.
3. **Stable and Open Move:** repeat on other side.

Reminders

- Begin with feet in the **Horse Stance, Center Position** (see **Posture,** page 14), with arms in front of the body as if holding a large ball. Fingertips face each other, without touching, at midline.
- Shift weight onto one foot as the other foot turns out to a 45-degree angle and arms open expressively.
- Head, trunk and pelvis rotate in direction of unweighted foot.
- Eyes gaze forward with the movement of the head, maintaining awareness of the periphery.
- Knee of the stable leg is bent and the weight is evenly distributed over entire sole of foot.
- Knee of the stable leg remains in alignment with the foot.
- Body remains in an upright position throughout the entire movement.

Benefits

- External hip rotation stretches the groin muscles, which can become tight with disuse.
- This movement increases range of motion and strength in the hip area, contributing to dynamic balance.
- Scapular muscles are activated, counteracting the flexed posture characteristic of older adults.
- Shoulder muscle activation against gravity promotes greater cardiovascular benefits.
- Expansion of the chest muscles to an open, extended posture can have a positive, emotional benefit.

Discussion

Start by learning the leg movements before adding the arms. Support should be used for people with balance and weight-shifting limitations. This is an excellent movement for patients with tight groin muscles or weakness in the hip muscles. Use this movement to start balance training. For those with a flexed posture, eventually add the arm movements. Try using this as an exercise with patients who have a history of depression.

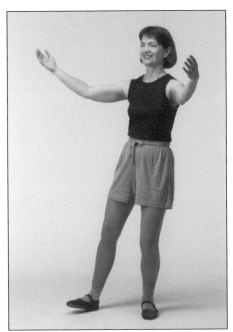

1. Stable and Open Move; arms open

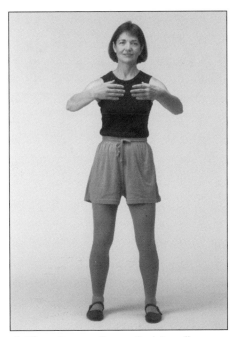

2. Horse Stance, Center Position; fingers at midline

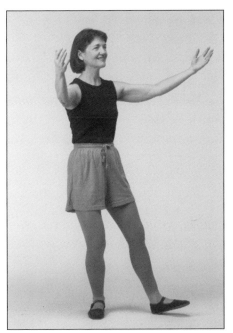

3. Stable and Open Move; arms open

Bear Rooting

Bear Rooting involves double limb weight shifting progressing to single limb stance.

Movements

1. **Horse Stance, Single-Limbed Position:** weight shifts 100 percent onto one foot. Forearms parallel to floor throughout entire movement.
2. **Horse Stance, Center Position.**
3. **Horse Stance, Single-Limbed Position:** weight shifts 100 percent onto the other foot.

Reminders

- Begin in the **Horse Stance, Center Position** (see **Posture**, page 14), with forearms parallel to floor.
- Knees remain flexed and the body upright as the weight shifts from one foot to the other.
- Knee of the stable leg remains in alignment with the foot.
- Knee of the stable leg is bent and the weight is evenly distributed over entire sole of foot.
- Body remains in an upright position throughout the entire movement. The tailbone maintains alignment with the heels.
- Unweighted foot lifts off the ground while the pelvis remains balanced.

"Separate the weight."
Benjamin Pang Jeng Lo

"If the weight of the whole body is resting on the right leg, then the right leg is substantial and the left leg is insubstantial and visa versa. If you cannot separate them, then the stance is not firm and can easily be thrown off balance."
Yang Cheng Fu

Benefits

- This movement demonstrates "rooting" in T'ai Chi practice.
- This movement helps establish a stable base of support and strengthens the thigh muscles.
- This is good training for advanced functional movements that incorporate balance, such as gait training and transfers.
- The flexed knees shift the weight to the lower extremity, making this an excellent load-bearing exercise.
- Weight is evenly distributed on the balls and heels of the feet, energetically connecting to the Earth *qi* through the *Yung Ch'uan* or "Bubbling Well" point, which is located in the middle of the sole of the foot, one-third anterior and two-thirds posterior, when the foot is in plantar flexion.

Discussion

Individuals with balance limitations and weak thigh muscles will benefit from this movement, but may need to start with support. Remember to include the breathing and posture instructions through all movements.

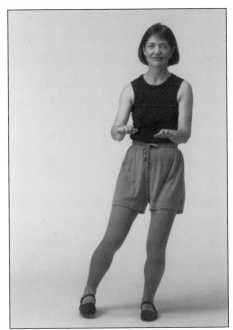

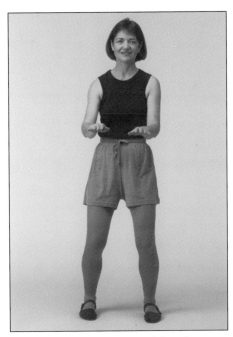

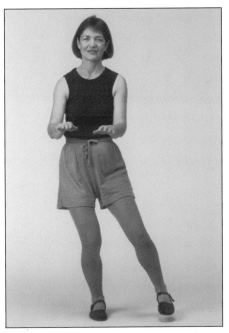

1. Horse Stance, Single-Limbed Position; forearms parallel to floor

2. Horse Stance, Center Position; forearms parallel to floor

3. Horse Stance, Single-Limbed Position; forearms parallel to floor

The 70/30 Stance

The **70/30 Stance** is an important position practiced throughout the T'ai Chi Form. It provides a wide base of support that maximizes stability throughout weight shifts. When the weight is forward, 70 percent is on the front foot and 30 percent is on the back foot. When the weight is on the back foot, it can support up to 100 percent of the weight.

Movements

1. **Stable and Open Position.**
2. **70/30 Stance, Back Position:** shift weight onto the diagonal foot and step directly forward, heel first, with the straight foot, maintaining hip-distance width. Keep 100 percent of the weight on the diagonal back foot. The back foot is at 45 degrees. Trunk and pelvis face the direction of the front foot.
3. **70/30 Stance, Forward Position:** shift forward until more weight is on the front foot (70 percent).
4. **Stable and Open Position** (other side).
5. **70/30 Stance, Back Position:** (other side) with 100 percent of the weight on the back foot.
6. **70/30 Stance, Forward Position:** (other side) with more weight on the front foot (70 percent).

Reminders

- Begin with **Stable and Open Move.** (See page 22)
- When stepping forward, step with the heel first, like walking.
- Pelvis stays in a neutral position throughout the movement.
- Pelvis faces the direction of the front foot.
- During all weight shifting, the knees maintain a flexed position.

- When shifting forward, the front knee maintains alignment with the foot.
- Knee of the front foot does not flex beyond the front toe.
- When shifting back, there is increased flexion of the hip and knee.
- Feet remain flat with weight evenly distributed over entire soles throughout the weight shift.
- Body remains in an upright position throughout the entire movement.
- Body remains at same height throughout the weight shifts. (avoid standing up when shifting the weight onto the back foot).

Benefits

- This movement provides good practice in anterior/posterior weight shifting. This is an important component of gait training.
- It promotes increased ankle range of motion and facilitates lengthening of the calf muscles.
- The thighs are strengthened as they work through a shortened range.

Discussion

This is an excellent precursor to gait training and advanced functional movements. The weight shifting in the flexed position facilitates increased load bearing and may be beneficial for increasing the bone density of the lower extremity.

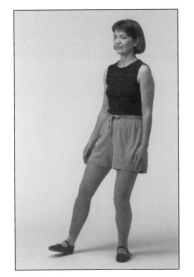

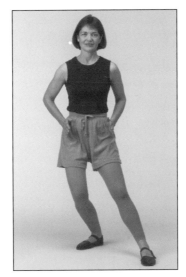

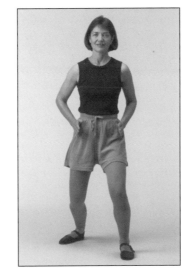

1. *Stable and Open Position*

2. *70/30 Stance, Back Position*

3. *70/30 Stance, Forward Position*

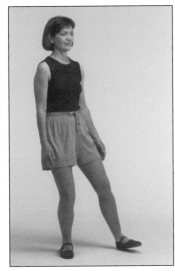

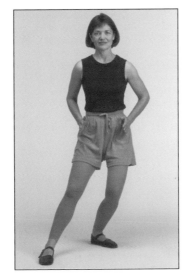

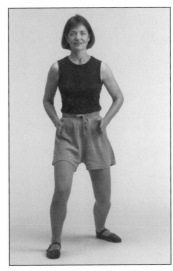

4. *Stable and Open Position*

5. *70/30 Stance, Back Position*

6. *70/30 Stance, Forward Position*

The Bear Walk

This Movement Pattern provides practice in the **70/30 Stance,** an important position repeated throughout the T'ai Chi Form.

Movements

1. **Stable and Open Position:** arms are relaxed at sides.
2. **70/30 Stance, Back Position:** shift weight onto the diagonal foot and step directly forward with the straight foot, maintaining hip-distance width. Keep 100 percent of the weight on the diagonal back foot. The back foot is at 45 degrees and the body facing forward in the direction of the front foot. Arms swing back.
3. **70/30 Stance, Forward Position:** shift forward until more weight is on the front foot (70 percent). Arms swing forward.
4.. **Stable and Open Position:** (other side) arms are relaxed at sides.
5. **70/30 Stance, Back Position:** (other side) with 100 percent of the weight on the back foot. Arms swing back.
6. **70/30 Stance, Forward Position:** (other side) with more weight on the front foot (70 percent). Arms swing forward.

Reminders

- Begin with **Stable and Open Move** (See page 22).
- See **70/30 Stance** (Page 26).
- Arms remain relaxed as they swing forward and back with the weight shift.

Benefits

- Arm movements activate the shoulder flexors in an anti-gravity position.
- Synchronizing the breath with the arms, inhaling as they are raised and exhaling as they are lowered, contributes to greater relaxation.

Discussion

See **70/30 Stance** (Page 26).
The anti-gravity arm movements are a good strengthening exercise for the upper extremity and can be used as a cardiac work out as well. When the arms swing further forward and back, they are called the "Crane Arms"

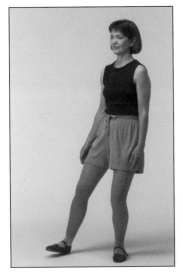

*1. Stable and Open Position;
arms relaxed at sides*

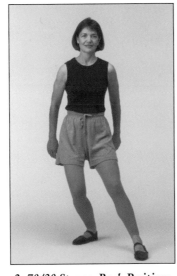

*2. 70/30 Stance, Back Position;
arms swing back*

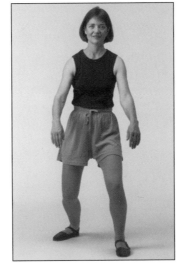

*3. 70/30 Stance, Forward
Position; arms swing forward*

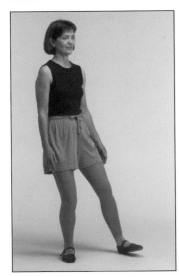

*4. Stable and Open Position;
arms relaxed at sides*

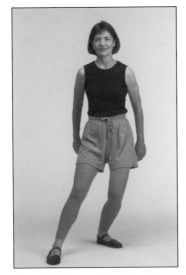

*5. 70/30 Stance, Back Position;
arms swing back*

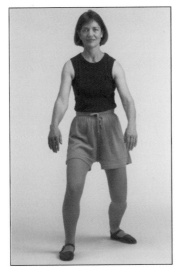

*6. 70/30 Stance, Forward
Position; arms swing forward*

The Movement Patterns of Section Two

The movements of this section involve rotation of the trunk and pelvis as a unit over the stable legs. There is currently no medical terminology to describe this action, which we call the T'ai Chi Fold. It represents a more advanced progression involving a separation of the lower and upper body.

The T'ai Chi Fold

The **T'ai Chi Fold** is a diagonal "fold" in loose clothing at the place where the hip joint forms a crease at the top of the femoral triangle. It is a key area of focus in the practice of T'ai Chi. This area is called the *Kwa*. This exercise involves "folding" and "sinking" into the *Kwa*.

Movements

1. **Horse Stance with T'ai Chi Fold:** rotate trunk and pelvis to one side.
2. **Horse Stance, Center Position:** rotate trunk and pelvis to center.
3. **Horse Stance with T'ai Chi Fold:** rotate trunk and pelvis to other side.

Reminders

- Begin in the **Horse Stance, Center Position** (see **Posture**, page 14).
- As trunk and pelvis rotate to one side, the weight will naturally shift more onto the foot of that side.
- Eyes gaze forward with the movement of the head, trunk and pelvis, maintaining awareness of the periphery.
- Both feet remain flat throughout entire movement
- Knees remain flexed and the body upright as the weight shifts more onto one foot.

- Knee maintains alignment with the foot of the more weighted leg.
- Shoulders maintain alignment over hips.
- Pelvis is relaxed in a neutral position with the tailbone in line with the heels

Benefits

- The movement of the pelvis over stable legs is a powerful wind-up motion in many sports activities.
- When done repetitively, it loosens that area and may increase circulation to the hip joint, which tends to have a poor blood supply.
- Loosening this area of the hip can influence balance control by widening the base of support and maintaining alignment of the hip, knee and foot.

Discussion

This represents a unique aspect of T'ai Chi that can be performed properly only after mastering the basics of Section One. The elements of the **T'ai Chi Fold** include: rooting, sinking, turning and weight shifting. Many people have not experienced rotation of the pelvis over stable legs.

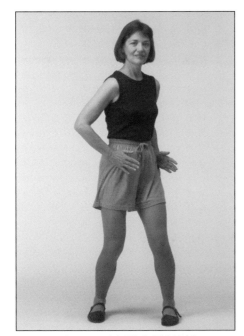

1. Horse Stance with T'ai Chi Fold

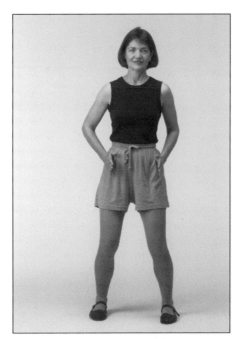

2. Horse Stance, Center Position

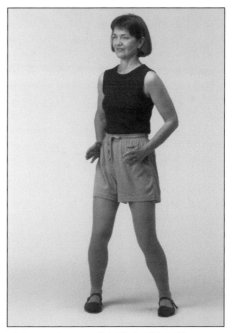

3. Horse Stance with T'ai Chi Fold

The Basic Bear

This is the most common T'ai Chi warm-up with the **T'ai Chi Fold**. It involves a double-stance weight shift as the trunk and pelvis rotate as a unit over the stable legs.

"Stand like a balance, rotate actively like a wheel."

Wang Tsung Yueh

Movements

1. **Horse Stance with T'ai Chi Fold:** rotate trunk and pelvis to one side. Arms swing in circular motion.
2. **Horse Stance, Center Position:** rotate trunk and pelvis to center. Arms swing in circular motion.
3. **Horse Stance with T'ai Chi Fold:** rotate trunk and pelvis to other side. Arms swing in circular motion.

Reminders

• See **T'ai Chi Fold** (page 30) for movement of the trunk and pelvis.
• Arms stay relaxed, swinging in a circular motion with the torso movement.

Benefits

• See **T'ai Chi Fold** (page 30).

Discussion

See **T'ai Chi Fold** (page 30). This rotation of the torso also is characteristic of the wind-up motion in swinging a golf club, batting a base ball and hitting a tennis ball.

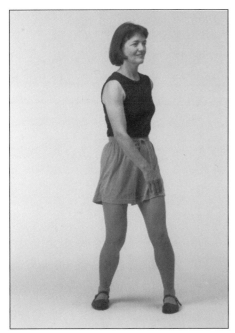 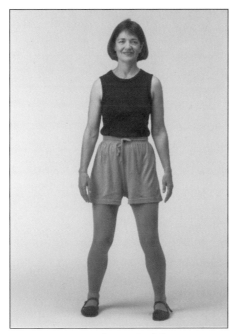 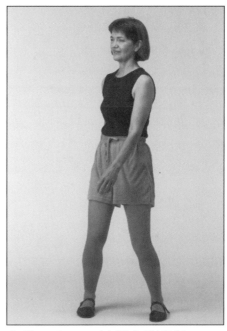

1. *Horse Stance with T'ai Chi Fold; arms swing in circular motion*

2. *Horse Stance, Center Position; arms relaxed at sides*

3. *Horse Stance with T'ai Chi Fold; arms swing in circular motion*

Holding the Moon

This is based on a *Qigong* exercise traditionally done standing, without trunk and pelvis rotation. This movement incorporates the trunk and pelvis rotation of the **T'ai Chi Fold** with the addition of a stable arm position.

"Upper and lower mutually follow."
Yang Cheng-Fu

"Keep your fingers naturally open, not too bent, not too straight, not too spread apart."
Chen Wei-Ming

Movements

1. **Horse Stance with T'ai Chi Fold:** rotate trunk and pelvis to one side with the arms in **Holding the Moon Position** in front of the body.
2. **Horse Stance, Center Position:** rotate trunk and pelvis to center maintaining position of arms.
3. **Horse Stance with T'ai Chi Fold:** rotate trunk and pelvis to the other side maintaining position of arms.

Reminders

- See **T'ai Chi Fold** (page 30) for movement of the trunk and pelvis.
- Position the arms in front of the body as if holding a large ball. Fingertips face each other, without touching, at midline.
- Thumbs point to each other forming the shape of a crescent moon.
- Arms and fingers remain in this position throughout the movement.
- Shoulders and elbows are relaxed and heavy.

Benefits:

- Hands are positioned at midline throughout the movement and act as a marker, helping reinforce proper positioning of the trunk over the pelvis.

Discussion:

See **T'ai Chi Fold** (page 30).

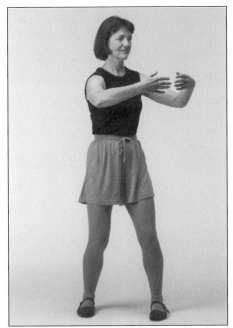

1. Horse Stance with T'ai Chi Fold; arms in Holding the Moon Position

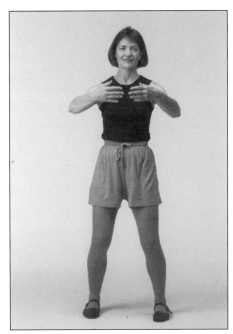

2. Horse Stance, Center Position; arms in Holding the Moon Position

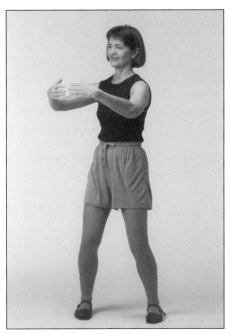

3. Horse Stance with T'ai Chi Fold; arms in Holding the Moon Position

Ski Move

The **T'ai Chi Fold** movement is done with the addition of yet another arm position.

Movements

1. **Horse Stance with T'ai Chi Fold:** rotate trunk and pelvis to one side as arms swing in opposition.
2. **Horse Stance, Center Position:** rotate trunk and pelvis to center with arms at sides.
3. **Horse Stance with T'ai Chi Fold:** rotate trunk and pelvis to other side as arms swing in opposition.

Reminders

- See **T'ai Chi Fold** (page 30) for movement of the trunk and pelvis.
- Arms now swing in opposition in a fashion similar to cross-country skiing.
- Relax shoulders and arms.

Benefits

- The reciprocal arm movement reinforces a natural pattern in ambulation and is often lacking in older adults.
- These arm movements support a deeper rotation of the pelvis.

Discussion

Adding arm movements associated with familiar activities such as walking or cross country skiing, allows the body to move through multiple joint movements in a coordinated fashion.

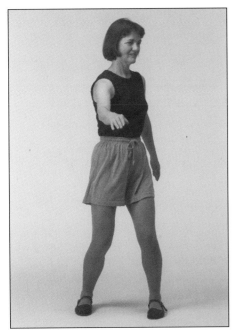

1. Horse Stance with T'ai Chi Fold; arms swing in opposition

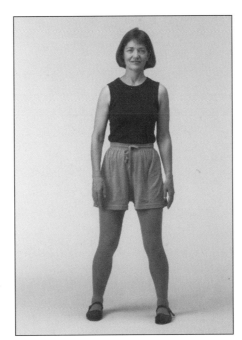

2. Horse Stance, Center Position; arms at sides

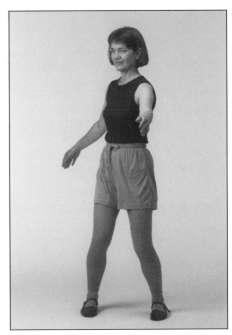

3. Horse Stance with T'ai Chi Fold; arms swing in opposition

The Movement Patterns of Section Three

These final movements are the most advanced in terms of balance and coordination.

The Flying Crane

This graceful movement involves balancing on one foot in a continuous weight-shifting pattern.

Movements

1. **Flying Crane Stance:** lift knee of unweighted leg to the front, raising arms at sides.
2. **Transition:** lower leg, lowering arms at sides.
3. **Flying Crane Stance:** shift weight and repeat movement on other leg.

Reminders

- Begin in the **Horse Stance, Center Position** (page 14), and move into the **Stable and Open Position** (see page 22).
- Shift weight onto the diagonal foot.
- When lifting the unweighted leg, keep the toes touching the ground for balance if necessary.
- Lower unweighted leg and position foot to the diagonal before shifting weight onto it.
- Pelvis maintains a neutral position with hip bones level throughout the entire movement.
- Knee of the stable leg remains bent throughout the movement.
- Knee of the stable leg remains in alignment with the foot.
- Unweighted leg is relaxed so that the lower leg dangles from the knee like a pendulum.
- Ankle of unweighted leg is relaxed.

- Arm movements are similar to **Crane Takes Flight** (see page 20) and can be performed with thumb and fingers touching as arms are raised.

Benefits

- Balancing on one foot in a continuous weight-shifting pattern improves balance and builds strength.
- This movement challenges the center of gravity, which in turn will improve both static and dynamic balance.

Discussion

The key is to maintain stability throughout the transitions in movement, with the "full" or weighted leg supporting the entire body, and the other leg completely "empty." Initially, some people will prefer to use support when balancing.

Keep the knee of the stable leg bent throughout the movement. Most people will tend to extend the knee as they raise their arms. It is important to keep the knee of the weighted leg aligned over the foot. This reduces stress on the knee.

People often hold their breath when their balance is challenged. This movement can be used to practice breathing while balancing. Inhale as arms are raised, exhale as they are lowered.

Remember, when moving, there is no place that doesn't move. When still, there is no place that isn't still."
Wu Yu Hsiang

"Expansion and contraction, opening and closing should be natural."
T'ai Chi Classics, author unknown

"Upper and lower mutually follow."
Yang Cheng Fu

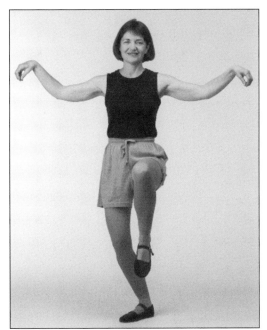

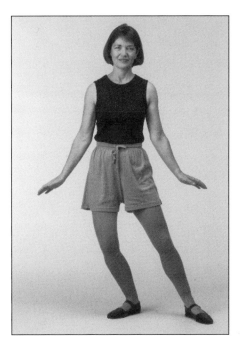

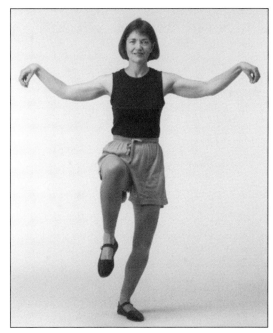

1. Flying Crane Stance; arms raised at sides

2. Transition; arms lowered at sides

3. Flying Crane Stance; arms raised at sides

The 70/30 Stance with the T'ai Chi Fold

This combines the **70/30 Stance** (see page 26) with the **T'ai Chi Fold** (see page 30). This is a complex Movement Pattern which is practiced throughout most T'ai Chi forms.

Movements

1. **70/30 Stance, Back Position with T'ai Chi Fold:** weight shifts back, the pelvis rotates toward the back leg.
2. **70/30 Stance, Forward Position:** weight shifts forward, the pelvis faces forward in the direction of the front leg.
3. **70/30 Stance, Back Position with T'ai Chi Fold** (other side).
4. **70/30 Stance, Forward Position** (other side).

Reminders

- Feet maintain shoulder width in the **70/30 Stance** (see page 26) as the body shifts back and forth.
- As the weight shifts back, the pelvis rotates toward the back leg. (see **T'ai Chi Fold**, page 30).
- As the pelvis rotates toward the back leg, the front knee maintains alignment with the front foot.
- As the weight shifts forward, the pelvis returns to neutral in the direction of the front leg.
- When shifting forward, the front knee maintains alignment with the foot.
- Knee of the front foot does not flex beyond the front toe.
- When shifting back, there is increased flexion of the back hip, knee and ankle.
- Feet remain flat with weight evenly distributed over entire soles throughout the weight shift.
- Body remains in an upright position throughout the entire movement.

- Body remains at same height throughout the weight shift (avoid standing up when shifting the weight onto the back foot).
- Head is "Suspended from Above" as the whole body relaxes and "sinks" throughout the movement.

Benefits

- This **70/30 Stance** promotes lengthening of the calf muscles and flexibility in the ankle joints.
- In addition to the anterior/posterior weight shift, the element of rotation is added to this movement.
- The movement of the pelvis over stable legs is a powerful wind-up motion in many sports activities.
- When done repetitively, it loosens that area and may increase circulation to the hip joint, which tends to have a poor blood supply.
- Loosening this area of the hip can influence balance control by widening the base of support and maintaining alignment of the hip, knee and foot.

Discussion

This movement includes the following basic components that are integral to traditional T'ai Chi practice. Body remains in an upright position, shoulders maintain alignment over hips. Both feet remain flat and firmly rooted. While turning or "folding" at the *Kwa*, or hip joint, the pelvis and trunk move as a unit.

Note: People often will tend to lead with the shoulders and twist the torso, thereby eliminating the action in the hips. Due to restrictions in mobility of the hips and ankles, people may also move the pelvis out of alignment, lean forward or to the side. The T'ai Chi Classics emphasize the importance of the unified movement of the trunk and pelvis as key to the practice of T'ai Chi.

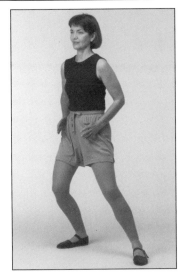

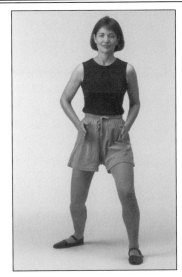

1. 70/30 Stance, Back Position with T'ai Chi Fold

2. 70/30 Stance, Forward Position

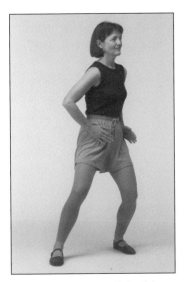

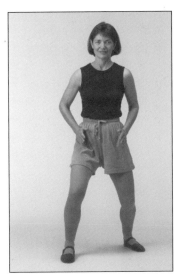

3. 70/30 Stance, Back Position with T'ai Chi Fold

4. 70/30 Stance, Forward Position

The Softball Pitch or Bowling Move

This combines the **70/30 Stance** with the **T'ai Chi Fold** and involves rotation of the trunk and pelvis. The arm movements combine those of the **Basic Bear** with those of the **Ski Move.**

"The motion should be rooted in the feet, released through the legs, guided by the torso, and expressed through the fingers."

Chang San Feng

Movements

1. **70/30 Stance, Back Position with T'ai Chi Fold:** weight shifts back, the pelvis rotates toward the back leg. Arms circle with rotation of trunk and pelvis.
2. **70/30 Stance, Forward Position:** weight shifts forward, the pelvis faces forward in the direction of the front leg. One arm swings forward, the other swings back.
3. **70/30 Stance, Back Position with T'ai Chi Fold** (repeat on other side).
4. **70/30 Stance, Forward Position**(repeat on other side)

Reminders

- See **70/30 Stance with the T'ai Chi Fold** (page 40).
- As the weight shifts back, the arms circle with the movement of the pelvis and trunk, imitating the **Basic Bear** arms (see page 32).
- As the weight shifts forward, the arms extend forward and back like the **Ski Move** (see page 36).

Benefits

- See **70/30 Stance with the T'ai Chi Fold** (page 40).
- In addition to the anterior/posterior weight shift, the element of rotation is added to this movement, along with arm swing. These complex moves benefit gait training and coordination.
- The reciprocal arm movement reinforces a natural pattern in ambulation that is often lacking in older adults.
- These arm movements support a deeper rotation of the pelvis.

Discussion

See **70/30 Stance with the T'ai Chi Fold** (page 40). Adding arm movements associated with familiar activities such as pitching a soft ball or bowling allows the body to move through multiple joint movements in a coordinated fashion.

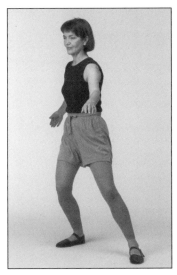

1. 70/30 Stance, Back Position
with T'ai Chi Fold; arms
swing in circular motion

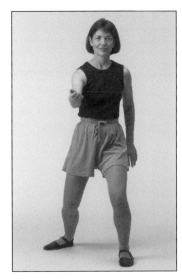

2. 70/30 Stance, Forward
Position; arms move in opposition

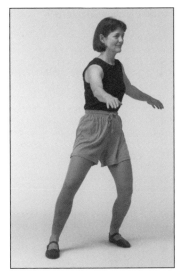

3. 70/30 Stance, Back Position
with T'ai Chi Fold; arms
swing in circular motion

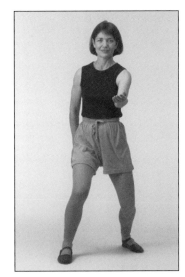

4. 70/30 Stance, Forward
Position; arms move in opposition

The Dancing Crane

This final Movement Pattern is a progression from the **Flying Crane** and requires the most joint range and muscle flexibility of the hip and groin.

Movements

1. **Dancing Crane Stance:** lift leg rotating externally as arms open expressively.
2. **Transition:** lower leg as arms move into **Holding the Moon Position.**
3. **Dancing Crane Stance:** Repeat movement on other side.

Reminders

- Begin in the **Horse Stance, Center Position** (see **Posture,** page 14).
- Move into the **Stable and Open** position (see page 22), and shift weight onto the diagonal foot.
- Weight is evenly distributed over entire sole of weighted foot.
- Knee of the stable leg remains bent throughout the movement.
- Knee of the stable leg remains in alignment with the foot.
- Unweighted leg is externally rotated and lifted to the diagonal keeping the foot and ankle relaxed. Foot extends beyond the knee in a kick position.
- Toes of the unweighted foot can touch the ground for balance if necessary.
- Pelvis faces forward and stays balanced.
- Body stays upright.
- Head turns to face the direction of the kick.
- Eyes gaze forward with the movement of the head, maintaining awareness of the periphery.

- Lower unweighted leg and position foot to the diagonal before shifting weight onto it.
- Arm movements begin in the **Holding the Moon Position** (see page 34) position and open expressively.

Benefits

- This movement exercises the center of gravity in preparation for actual challenges in balance.
- Adding the arm movements contributes to both cardiovascular and emotional benefits.

Discussion

Like the **Flying Crane** (see page 38), this movement challenges dynamic balance. In contrast, the "empty" leg is externally rotated and abducted, lengthening the groin muscles. It is important to keep the knee of the weighted leg aligned over the foot. This reduces stress on the knee.

The arm movements stretch the pectoralis muscles and activate the scapular muscles, promoting more extension and improved posture.

"The body is like a floating cloud."
Cheng Man Ching

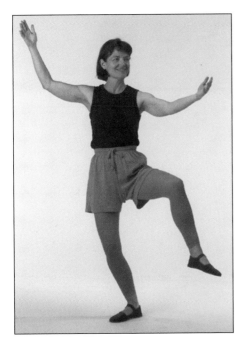

1. Dancing Crane Stance; arms open expressively

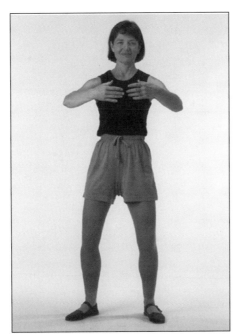

2. Transition: arms Holding the Moon

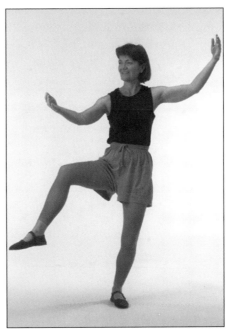

3. Dancing Crane Stance; arms open expressively

CHAPTER THREE

The T'ai Chi Fundamentals Form

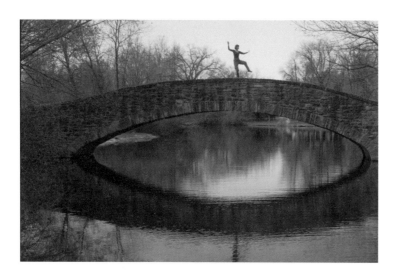

Description

This chapter includes reminders for performing the **Movements** of the Fundamentals Form, targets the **Corresponding Movement Patterns**, and includes a description of the **Modifications from Traditional Yang Style T'ai Chi.**

The T'ai Chi Fundamentals Form progresses from simple to more complex movements and eliminates some of the more difficult elements from the traditional form. The arm movements are simplified, and many movements are repeated bilaterally.

Each section of the T'ai Chi Fundamentals Form represents a progression in difficulty from the Movement Patterns in that section. The earlier sections may provide a complete and challenging program for many individuals.

Names of Movements

Section One	**Section Two**	**Section Three**
Preparation	Repulse the Monkey	Snake Slides Down
Beginning	Cloud Hands	Golden Pheasant
Ward Off	Single Whip	Stands on one Leg
Press		Separate Arms and Kick
Push		Brush Knee and Twist
Ward Off		Punch
Press		Withdraw and Push
Push		Cross Hands
		Closing

T'ai Chi Fundamentals Form: Section One

Corresponding Movement Patterns:

Posture and Breathing
Arm Swinging
Crane Takes Flight
Stable and Open Move
Bear Rooting
Bear Walk

Preparation

Movements

1. **Begin with feet in "V" position:** with body upright and relaxed, with heels together at a 45 degree angle and weight evenly distributed between the feet.
   Arms relaxed: hanging at sides.
2. Shift weight 100 percent onto right foot, knee aligned over foot. Move left foot directly to side, shoulder width, pointing forward.
3. Shift weight 100 percent onto left foot, knee aligned over foot. As weight shifts, trunk and pelvis rotate to the right diagonal.
4. **Move into Horse Stance, Center Position:** Rotate trunk and pelvis back to center, pivoting on right heel, bringing right foot parallel to the left foot. Both feet point forward, hip-distance apart. Shift weight to center, with weight evenly distributed, knees slightly bent and aligned over feet.
   Arms in Energetic Position: relaxed at sides, fingers facing down and slightly forward. Elbows slightly bent, wrists extended in neutral position.

Corresponding Movement Pattern

- **Horse Stance, Center Position** (see **Posture**, page 14).
- **Open and Stable Move** (see page 22).

Modifications from Traditional Yang Style

- Ending position with knees slightly bent.

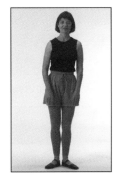
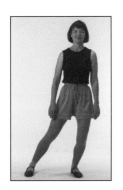
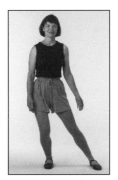
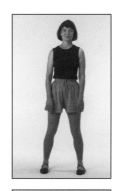

Front View:
Mirror Image

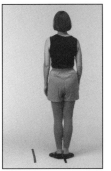
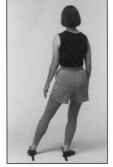
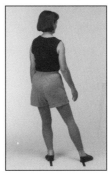
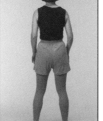

Back View:
Movements as described

1. Feet in "V" Position; arms relaxed at sides

2. Left foot points forward, weight 100 percent on right foot

3. Left foot points forward, weight 100 percent on left foot

4. Feet in Horse Stance, Center Position; arms in Energetic Position

Beginning

Movements

1. **Begin in Horse Stance, Center Position:** both feet point forward, hip-distance apart, weight evenly distributed, knees slightly bent and aligned over feet.
   Arms in Energetic Position: relaxed at sides with elbows slightly bent, wrists extended in neutral position. Fingers point down and forward.
2. **Raise arms:** to shoulder height and width, wrists flexed, fingers pointing down.
3. **Bend elbows:** slightly, extending wrists into neutral position, fingers point forward, palms face the ground. Draw hands toward shoulders, flexing elbows and wrists. Upper arms move next to body, shoulders relaxed, fingers point forward, palms face ground.
4. **Lower wrists and arms:** extend wrists into neutral position.
5. **End in Horse Stance, Center Position** (same as above).
   Arms in Energetic Position (same as above).

Corresponding Movement Pattern

- **Horse Stance, Center Position** (see **Posture,** page 14).

Modifications from Traditional Yang Style

- Ending position with knees slightly bent.

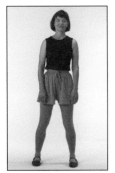
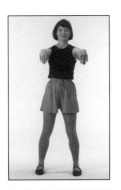
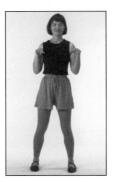
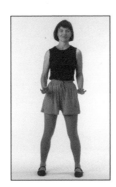
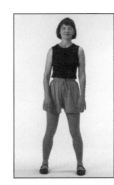

Front View:
Mirror Image

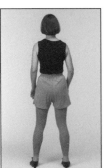
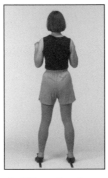
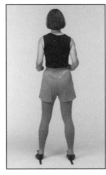
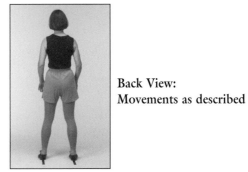

Back View:
Movements as described

1. Horse Stance; arms in Energetic Position

2. Arms raised to shoulder height and width

3. Elbows bend, upper arms at sides, fingers point forward

4. Lower wrists

5. Horse Stance; arms in Energetic Position

Ward Off (Left)

Movements

1. **Begin in Horse Stance, Center Position**: both feet point forward, hip-distance apart, weight evenly distributed, knees slightly bent and aligned over feet.
Arms in Energetic Position: relaxed at sides with elbows slightly bent, wrists in neutral position, fingers point down and forward.

2. **Move feet into Stable and Open Position**: shift weight 100 percent onto left leg. Rotate trunk and pelvis to right diagonal pivoting right heel to the diagonal. Left knee stays aligned over foot.
Simultaneously move arms into Holding Ball.
Position: move right hand to chest height facing down, move left hand to belly height facing up.

3. **Move feet into 70/30 Stance, Back Position**: shift weight 100 percent onto right foot. Step directly forward with left foot maintaining a hip-distance width stance.
Arms remain in Holding Ball Position.

4. **Move feet into 70/30 Stance, Forward Position**: shift weight forward onto the left foot (70 percent) with the knees maintaining a flexed position. Front knee maintains alignment with the front foot and does not move beyond the toes. During weight shift, the pelvis and trunk move to a neutral position, facing forward in the direction of the left foot. Feet are hip-distance apart with the left foot pointing forward and right foot to the diagonal. Both feet are flat.

Simultaneously move arms into Ward Off, Left Position: raise left arm so that the palm faces the chest. Right arm drops next to right hip with elbow slightly bent, wrists in neutral position fingers point down and slightly forward.

Corresponding Movement Patterns
- **Horse Stance** (see **Posture,** page 14).
- **Stable and Open Position** (see page 22).
- **70/30 Stance** (see page 26).

Modifications from Traditional Yang Style
- In the transition from **Beginning** to **Left Ward Off,** the right foot is moved to the diagonal, rather than perpendicular to the left foot, thereby eliminating the heel pivot of the back foot during the forward weight shift into the **70/30 Stance.**

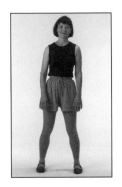
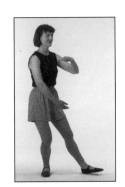
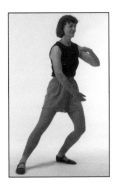
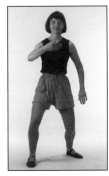

Front View:
Mirror Image

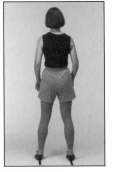
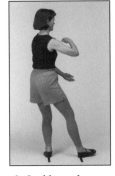
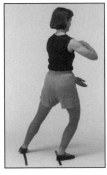
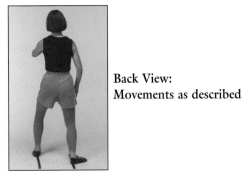

Back View:
Movements as described

*1. Horse Stance;
arms in Energetic
Position*

*2. Stable and
Open Stance; arms
in Holding Ball
Position*

*3. 70/30 Stance,
Back Position;
arms in Holding
Ball, Position*

*4. 70/30 Stance,
Forward Position;
arms in Ward-
Off, Left Position*

Press (Left)

Movements

1. **Begin in 70/30 Stance, Forward Position:** with more weight forward (70 percent) on the left foot. The front knee does not move beyond the front toe. Pelvis and trunk are in a neutral position, facing forward in the direction of the left foot. Feet are hip-distance width with the left foot pointing forward and right foot to the diagonal. Both feet are flat.
   Arms in Ward Off, Left Position: the left palm faces the chest; right elbow slightly bent, wrist in neutral position, fingers pointing down and forward.

2. **Move into 70/30 Stance Back Position:** shift 100 percent of the weight onto the right foot. Pelvis and trunk in neutral facing forward.
   Simultaneously bend right elbow: while shifting back, palm faces forward. Left elbow lowers slightly.

3. **Move into 70/30 Stance, Forward Position:** shift forward bringing most of the weight (70 percent) onto the left foot.
   Simultaneously move arms into Press Position: Left palm faces the chest, right palm presses lightly into wrist and base of left palm.

Corresponding Movement Pattern

- **70/30 Stance** (see page 26).

Modifications from Traditional Yang Style

- The movements are all done facing the direction of the **Beginning** position.
- There is no turning of the torso or folding of the *Kwa*.
- The back heel pivot is eliminated.

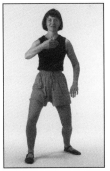
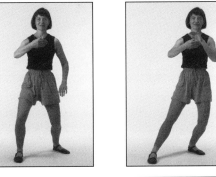
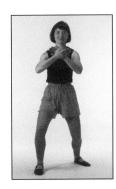

Front View:
Mirror Image

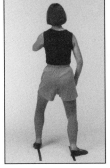
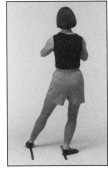
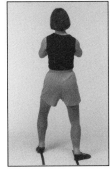

Back View:
Movements as described

*1. 70/30 Stance,
Forward Position;
arms in Ward
Off, Left Position*

*2. 70/30 Stance,
Back Position;
right elbow bent*

*3. 70/30 Stance,
Forward Position;
arms in Press
Position*

Push (Left)

Movements

1. **Begin in 70/30 Stance, Forward Position:** with more weight forward (70 percent) on the left foot. Front knee does not move beyond the front toe. Pelvis and trunk are in a neutral position, facing forward in the direction of the left foot. Feet are hip-distance width with the left foot pointing forward and the right foot to the diagonal. Both feet are flat.
   Arms in Press Position: left palm faces the chest; right palm presses lightly into base of left palm at the wrist.

2. **Move into 70/30 Stance, Back Position:** shift 100 percent of the weight onto the right foot, pelvis and trunk in neutral facing forward.
   Simultaneously move arms into Push Position: while shifting back, lower both elbows bringing the forearms parallel to each other, both palms face forward and slightly down.

3. **Move into 70/30 Stance, Forward Position:** shift forward bringing most of the weight (70 percent) onto the left foot.
   Arms remain in Push Position: parallel to each other, elbows heavy, wrists neutral, palms facing forward and slightly down.

Corresponding Movement Pattern

- **70/30 Stance** (see page 26).

Modifications from Traditional Yang Style

- The movements are all done facing the direction of the original starting position.

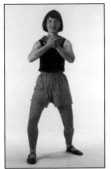 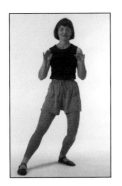

Front View:
Mirror Image

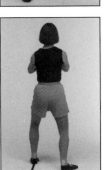 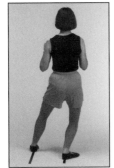 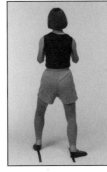

Back View:
Movements as described

1. 70/30 Stance,
Forward Position;
arms in Press
Position

2. 70/30 Stance,
Back Position;
arms in Push
Position

3. 70/30 Stance,
Forward Position;
arms in Push
Position

Ward Off (Right)

Movements

1. **Begin in 70/30 Stance, Forward Position:** with more weight forward (70 percent) on the left foot. Front knee does not move beyond the front toe. Pelvis and trunk are in a neutral position, facing forward in the direction of the left foot. Feet are hip-distance width with the left foot pointing forward and right foot to the diagonal. Both feet are flat.

    Arms in Push Position: arms remain parallel to each other, elbows heavy, wrists neutral, palms facing forward and slightly down.

2. **Diagonal Transition Position:** shift weight 100 percent onto right foot. Pelvis and trunk rotate to the left, pivoting on left heel, turn left foot to left diagonal. Right knee stays in alignment with foot.

    Simultaneously move arms into Holding Ball Position: left palm is chest height facing down, right palm is belly height facing up.

3. **Move into 70/30 Stance, Back Position:** shift weight 100 percent onto left foot. Step forward with right foot into **70/30 Stance**. Left knee stays in alignment with foot.

    Arms remain in Holding Ball Position: left palm is chest height facing down, right palm is belly height facing up.

4. **Move into 70/30 Stance, Forward Position:** shift weight forward onto the right foot (70 percent) with the knees maintaining a flexed position. Front knee maintains alignment with the front foot and does not move beyond the toes. As weight shifts, pelvis and trunk move to a neutral position, facing forward in the direction of the right foot. Feet are hip-distance apart with the right foot pointing forward and left foot to the diagonal. Both feet are flat.

Simultaneously move arms into Ward Off, Right Position: right palm faces the chest. Left arm drops next to left hip with elbow slightly bent, wrist in neutral position; fingers point down and slightly forward.

Corresponding Movement Pattern

- **70/30 Stance** (see page 26).

Modifications From Traditional Yang Style

- The transition resembles the transition from **Brush Knee and Twist Left** to **Brush Knee and Twist Right.**
- The left foot is moved to the diagonal rather than perpendicular to the right foot, thereby eliminating the heel pivot on the back foot.

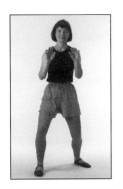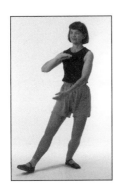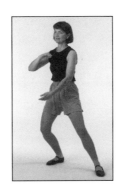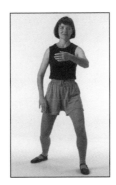

Front View:
Mirror Image

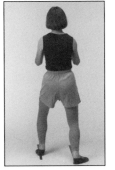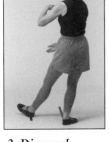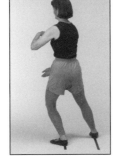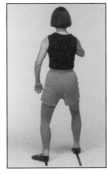

Back View:
Movements as described

1. 70/30 Stance,
Forward Position;
arms in Push
Position

2. Diagonal
Transition
Position; arms in
Holding Ball
Position

3. 70/30 Stance,
Back Position;
arms in Holding
Ball, Position

4. 70/30, Stance,
Forward Position;
arms in Ward
Off, Right
Position

The following Press and Push movements are identical to the those described on the preceding pages. The right foot is forward instead of the left foot.

Press (Right)

Movements

1. **Begin in 70/30 Stance, Forward Position:** with more weight forward (70 percent) on the right foot. Front knee does not move beyond the front toe. Pelvis and trunk are in a neutral position, facing forward in the direction of the right foot. Feet are shoulder width, with the right foot pointing forward and the left foot to the diagonal. Both feet are flat.
   Arms in Ward Off, Right Position: right palm faces the chest. Left elbow slightly bent, wrists in neutral position; fingers point down and slightly forward.
2. **Move into 70/30 Stance, Back Position:** shift 100 percent of the weight into the left foot, pelvis and trunk in neutral position, facing forward.
   Simultaneously bend left elbow while shifting back, palm faces forward; right elbow lowers slightly.
3. **Move into 70/30 Stance, Forward Position:** shift forward bringing most of the weight onto the right foot (70 percent).
   Simultaneously move arms into Press Position: right palm faces the chest. Left palm presses lightly on wrist and base of right palm.

Corresponding Movement Pattern

- **70/30 Stance** (see page 26).

Modifications From Traditional Yang Style

- The movements are all done facing the direction of the **Beginning** position.
- There is no turning of the torso or folding of the *Kwa*.

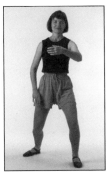 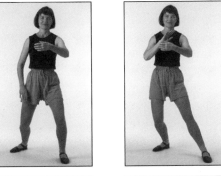 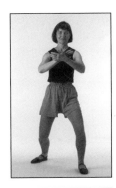

Front View:
Mirror Image

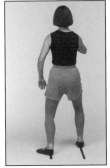 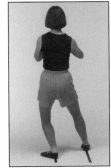 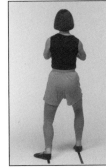

Back View:
Movements as described

1. *70/30 Stance,*
Forward Position;
arms in Ward
Off, Right
Position

2. *70/30 Stance,*
Back Position; left
elbow bent

3. *70/30 Stance,*
Forward Position;
arms in Press
Position

Push (Right)

Movements

1. **Begin in 70/30 Stance, Forward Position:** with more weight forward (70 percent) on the right foot. The front knee does not move beyond the front toe. Pelvis and trunk are in a neutral position, facing forward in the direction of the right foot. Feet are shoulder width with the right foot pointing forward and left foot to the diagonal. Both feet are flat.
   Arms in Press Position: right palm faces the chest. Left palm presses lightly into base of right palm at the wrist.
2. **Move into 70/30 Stance, Back Position:** shift 100 percent of the weight onto the left foot. Pelvis and trunk are in neutral position, facing forward.
   Simultaneously move arms into Push Position: while shifting back, lower both elbows bringing the forearms parallel to each other. Both palms face forward and slightly down.
3. **Move into 70/30 Stance, Forward Position:** shift forward bringing most of the weight (70 percent) onto the right foot.
   Arms remain in Push Position: arms remain parallel to each other, elbows heavy, wrists neutral, palms facing forward and slightly down.

Corresponding Movement Pattern

- **70/30 Stance** (see page 26).

Modifications from Traditional Yang Style

- The movements are all done facing the direction of the **Beginning** position.

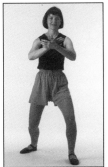 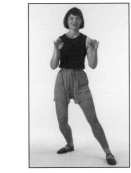 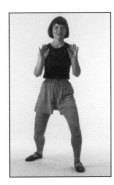

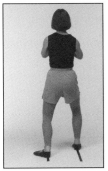 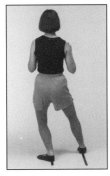 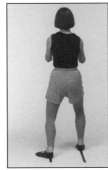

Front View:
Mirror Image

Back View:
Movements as described

*1. 70/30 Stance,
Forward Position;
arms in Press
Position*

*2. 70/30 Stance,
Back Position;
arms in Push
Position*

*3. 70/30 Stance,
Forward Position;
arms in Push
Position*

Step Forward

Movements

1. **Begin in 70/30 Stance, Forward Position:** with more weight (70 percent) on the right foot.
   Arms in Push Position: arms parallel to each other, elbows heavy, wrists neutral, palms facing forward and slightly down.
2. **Move into Horse Stance, Center Position:** shift weight 100 percent onto right foot. Bring left foot parallel to the right foot, both feet pointing forward, shoulder width apart. Shift weight 50 percent onto left foot so that weight is evenly distributed between both feet, knees slightly bent.
   Arms remain in Push Position: arms remain parallel to each other, elbows heavy, wrists neutral, palms facing forward and slightly down.

Corresponding Movement Pattern

- **70/30 Stance** (see page 26).
- **Bear Rooting** (see page 24).

Modifications from Yang Style

- The move ends with the feet in the **Horse Stance**.

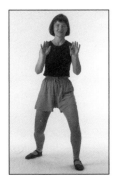

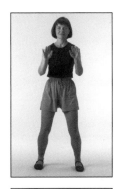

Front View:
Mirror Image

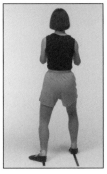

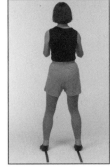

Back View:
Movements as described

1. 70/30 Stance,
Forward Position;
arms in Push
Position

2. Horse Stance,
Center Position;
arms in Push
Position

T'ai Chi Fundamentals Form: Section Two

Corresponding Movement Patterns:

All from Section One
Basic Bear
Holding the Moon
Ski Move

Repulse the Monkey, Trunk and Arm Movements

Movements

1. **Begin in Horse Stance, Center Position.**
   Arms in Push Position: arms parallel to each other, elbows heavy, wrists neutral, palms facing forward and slightly down.
2. **Move to Horse Stance with T'ai Chi Fold:** rotate pelvis and trunk to right diagonal as weight shifts more onto right foot.
   Simultaneously move arms to Repulse Monkey, Open Position: drop right arm to hip, palm facing forward. Then swing arm out to side, shoulder height, palm facing forward as left arm extends to front at shoulder height, palm facing down.
3. **Move arms to Repulse Monkey, Line-Up Position:** bend right elbow, fingers pointing forward as left palm turns to face up.
4. **Move to Horse Stance, Center Position:** rotate pelvis and trunk to neutral, facing forward as weight shifts to be evenly distributed on both feet.
   Simultaneously move arms to Repulse Monkey, Push Position: lower right elbow to front of body, wrist is neutral, palm facing forward and slightly down, as left hand drops to thigh, palm facing up and forward.

Repeat above movement to left as follows:

5. **Move to Horse Stance with T'ai Chi Fold:** rotate pelvis and trunk to left diagonal as weight shifts more onto left foot.
   Simultaneously move arms to Repulse Monkey, Open Position: swing left arm out to side, shoulder height, palm facing forward as right arm extends to front at shoulder height, palm facing down.
6. **Move arms to Repulse Monkey, Line-Up Position:** bend left elbow, fingers pointing forward as right palm turns up.
7. **Move to Horse Stance, Center Position:** rotate pelvis and trunk to neutral, facing forward as weight shifts to be evenly distributed on both feet.
   Simultaneously move arms to Repulse Monkey, Push Position: lower left elbow to front of body, wrist is neutral, palm facing forward and slightly down, as right hand drops to thigh, palm facing up and forward.

Corresponding Movement Pattern

- **Horse Stance** (see **Posture,** page 14).
- **T'ai Chi Fold** (see page 30).
- **Ski Move** (see page 36).

Modifications from Yang Style

- The feet remain in the **Horse Stance** throughout the entire movement.
- The trunk and arm movements are repeated alone.

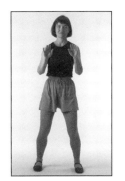
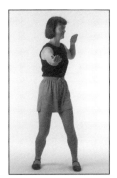
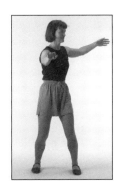
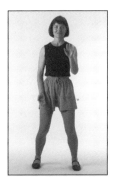
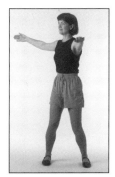
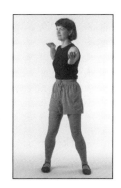
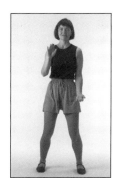

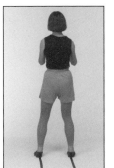
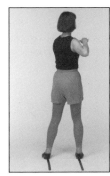
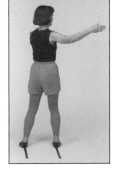
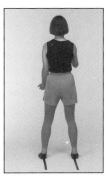
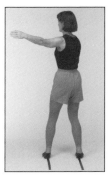
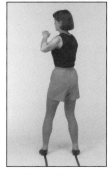
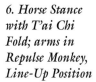
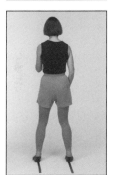

1. Horse Stance, Center Position; arms in Push Position

2. Horse Stance with T'ai Chi Fold; arms in Repulse Monkey, Open Position

3. Horse Stance with T'ai Chi Fold; arms in Repulse Monkey, Line-Up Position

4. Horse Stance, Center Position; arms in Repulse Monkey, Push Position

5. Horse Stance with T'ai Chi Fold; arms in Repulse Monkey, Open Position

6. Horse Stance with T'ai Chi Fold; arms in Repulse Monkey, Line-Up Position

7. Horse Stance, Center Position; arms in Repulse Monkey, Push Position

Repulse the Monkey, Right with Arm and Leg Movements

The trunk and arm movements are identical to those on the preceding page.

Movements

1. **Begin in Horse Stance, Center Position.**
   Arms in Repulse Monkey, Push Position: left elbow in front of body, wrist neutral, palm facing forward and slightly down. Right hand at thigh, palm facing up and forward.

2. **Move to Horse Stance with T'ai Chi Fold:** rotate pelvis and trunk to right diagonal as weight shifts 100 percent onto right foot.
   Simultaneously move arms to Repulse Monkey, Open Position: swing right arm out to side, shoulder height, palm facing forward as left arm extends to front at shoulder height, palm facing down.

3. **Move to Stagger Step, Forward Position:** step back with left foot, toes first, facing directly forward, parallel to and behind right foot, slightly narrower than shoulder width. Trunk and pelvis at right diagonal with tailbone in alignment with left heel.
   Simultaneously move arms to Repulse Monkey, Line-Up Position: simultaneously bend right elbow, fingers pointing forward. Turn left palm up.

4. **Move to Stagger Step, Back Position:** shift weight 100 percent onto left foot. Rotate pelvis and trunk to forward position.
   Simultaneously move arms into Repulse Monkey, Push Position: lower right elbow to front of body, wrist neutral, palm facing forward and slightly down, as left hand drops to thigh, palm facing up and forward.

Corresponding Movement Pattern

- **T'ai Chi Fold** (see page 30).
- **Ski Move** (see page 36).

Modifications from Yang Style

- None

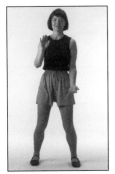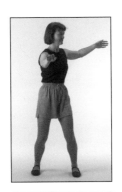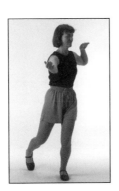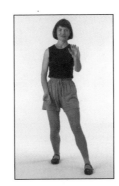

Front View:
Mirror Image

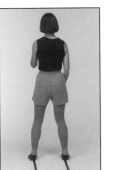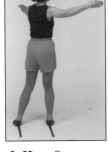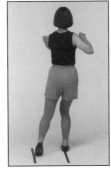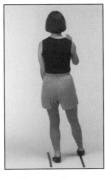

Back View:
Movements as described

1. Horse Stance, Center Position; arms in Repulse Monkey, Push Position

2. Horse Stance with T'ai Chi Fold; arms in Repulse Monkey, Open Position

3. Stagger Step, Front Position; arms in Repulse Monkey Line-Up Position

4. Stagger Step, Back Position; arms in Repulse Monkey Push Position

Repulse the Monkey, Left with Arm and Leg Movements

This movement is identical to the preceding movement except that it is performed turning to the left.

Movements

1. **Begin in Stagger Step, Back Position:** weight 100 percent on left foot, parallel to and behind right foot. Feet slightly narrower than shoulder width. Both feet face forward; pelvis and trunk face forward.
   Arms in Repulse Monkey, Push Position: right elbow bent in front of body, wrist neutral, palm facing forward and slightly down. Left hand at left thigh, palm facing up and forward.

2. **Move to Horse Stance with T'ai Chi Fold:** rotate pelvis and trunk to left diagonal.
   Simultaneously move arms to Repulse Monkey, Open Position: swing left arm out to side, shoulder height, palm facing forward as right arm extends to front, palm facing down.

3. **Move to Stagger Step, Forward Position:** step back with right foot, toes first, facing directly forward, parallel to and behind left foot, slightly narrower than shoulder width. Trunk and pelvis at left diagonal with tailbone in alignment with left heel.
   Simultaneously move arms to Repulse Monkey, Line-Up Position: bend left elbow, fingers pointing forward as right palm turns up.

4. **Move to Stagger Step, Back Position:** shift weight 100 percent onto right foot parallel to and behind left foot. Feet are slightly narrower than shoulder width. Rotate pelvis and trunk to neutral position. Both feet face forward. Pelvis and trunk face forward.
   Simultaneously move arms into Repulse Monkey, Push Position: lower left elbow to front of body, wrist neutral, palm facing forward and slightly down, as right hand drops to thigh, palm facing up and forward.

Corresponding Movement Pattern

- **T'ai Chi Fold** (see page 30).
- **Ski Move** (see page 36).

Modifications from Yang Style

- None

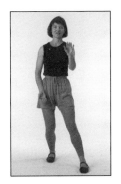 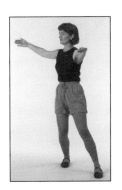 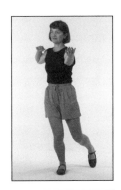 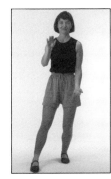

Front View:
Mirror Image

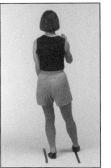 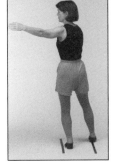 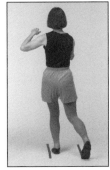 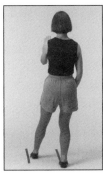

Back View:
Movements as described

1. Horse Stance, Center Position; arms in Repulse Monkey, Push Position

2. Horse Stance with T'ai Chi Fold; arms in Repulse Monkey, Open Position

3. Stagger Step, Forward Position; arms in Repulse Monkey, Line-Up Position

4. Stagger Step, Back Position; arms in Repulse Monkey, Push Position

Repulse the Monkey Right, to Horse Stance

The arm movements are identical to Repulse Monkey trunk and arm movements.

Movements

1. **Begin in Stagger Step, Back Position:** weight 100 percent on right foot, parallel to and behind left foot; feet slightly narrower than shoulder width; both feet facing forward. Pelvis and trunk face forward.
   Arms in Repulse Monkey, Push Position: left elbow bent at front of body, wrist neutral, palm facing forward and slightly down. Right hand at right thigh, palm facing up and forward.

2. **Move to Stagger Step, Back Position with T'ai Chi Fold:** rotate pelvis and trunk to right diagonal.
   Simultaneously move arms to Repulse Monkey, Open Position: swing right arm out to side, shoulder height, palm facing forward as left arm extends to front at shoulder height, palm facing down.

3. **Move into Horse Stance with T'ai Chi Fold:** move left foot back, toes first, parallel to the right foot, both feet pointing forward, hip-distance apart, weight 100 percent on right foot. Trunk and pelvis facing right diagonal with tailbone in alignment with right heel.
   Simultaneously move arms to Repulse Monkey, Line-Up Position: bend right elbow, fingers pointing forward as left palm turns up.

4. **Move into Horse Stance, Center Position:** shift weight evenly onto both feet. Rotate pelvis and trunk to forward position.
   Simultaneously move arms to Repulse Monkey, Push Position: lower right elbow to front of body, wrist neutral, palm facing forward and slightly down as left arm drops to hip, palm facing forward and up.

Corresponding Movement Pattern

- **T'ai Chi Fold** (see page 30).
- **Ski Move** (see page 36).

Modifications from Yang Style

- The movement ends with feet in the **Horse Stance**.

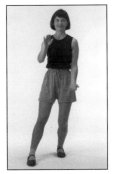
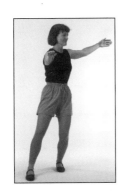
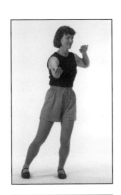
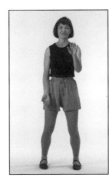

Front View:
Mirror Image

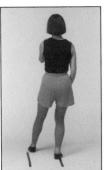
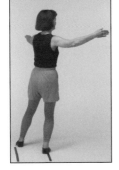
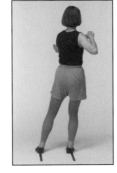
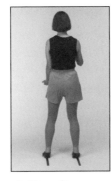

Back View:
Movements as described

*1. Stagger Step,
Back Position;
arms in Repulse
Monkey, Push
Position*

*2. Stagger Step,
Back Position
with T'ai Chi
Fold; arms in
Repulse Monkey,
Open Position*

*3. Horse Stance
with T'ai Chi
Fold; arms in
Line-Up Position*

*4. Horse Stance,
Center Position;
arms in Repulse
Monkey, Push
Position*

Cloud Hands, Trunk and Arm Movements

Movements

1. **Begin in Horse Stance, Center Position.**
   Arms in Repulse Monkey, Push Position: right elbow at front of body, wrists neutral, palms facing forward and slightly down. Left hand at thigh, palm facing forward and up.

2. **Move to Horse Stance with T'ai Chi Fold:** rotate pelvis and trunk to left diagonal as weight shifts more onto left foot.
   Simultaneously move arms into Holding the Ball Position: left hand chest height, palm facing down; right hand belly height, palm facing up.

3. **Move arms to Cloud Hands Position:** raise right hand on inside, palm facing chest as left hand lowers on outside, palm facing belly.
   Then move to Horse Stance, Center Position: rotate pelvis and trunk to center. Shift weight to the center, evenly distributed between both feet.

4. **Move to Horse Stance with T'ai Chi Fold:** rotate pelvis and trunk to right diagonal as weight shifts more onto right foot.
   Simultaneously move arms into Holding the Ball Position: right hand chest height, palm facing down; left hand belly height, palm facing up.

5. **Move arms to Cloud Hands Position:** raise left hand on inside, palm facing chest; lower right hand on outside, palm facing belly.
   Then move to Horse Stance, Center Position: rotate pelvis and trunk to center. Shift weight to the center, evenly distributed between both feet.

6. **Move to Horse Stance with T'ai Chi Fold:** rotate pelvis and trunk to left diagonal as weight shifts more onto left foot.
   Simultaneously move arms into Holding the Ball Position: left hand chest height, palm facing down; right hand belly height, palm facing up.

Corresponding Movement Pattern

- **T'ai Chi Fold** (see page 30).
- **Holding Moon** (see page 34).

Modifications from Yang Style

- Initially, the trunk and arm movements are repeated alone.

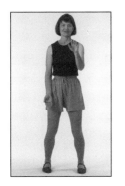 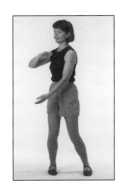 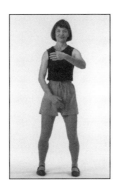 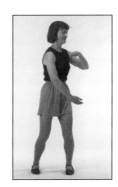 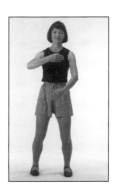 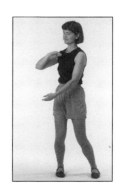

Front View:
Mirror Image

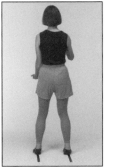 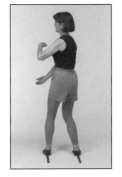 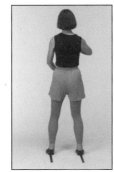 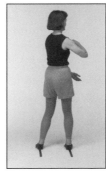 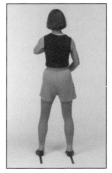 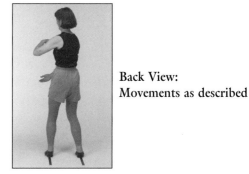

Back View:
Movements as described

1. Horse Stance; arms in Repulse Monkey, Push Position

2. Horse Stance with T'ai Chi Fold; arms in Holding the Ball Position

3. Horse Stance; arms in Cloud Hands Position

4. Horse Stance with T'ai Chi Fold; arms in Holding the Ball Position

5. Horse Stance; arms in Cloud Hands Position

6. Horse Stance with T'ai Chi Fold; arms in Holding the Ball Position

Cloud Hands, Arm and Leg Movements

The arm movements are identical to the preceding movements.

Movements

1. **Begin in Horse Stance with T'ai Chi Fold:** pelvis and trunk at left diagonal with more weight on left foot.
   Arms in Holding the Ball Position: left hand chest height, palm facing down, right hand belly height, palm facing up.
2. **Move to Wide Horse Stance with T'ai Chi Fold:** shift weight 100 percent onto left foot. Place flat right foot further out to right side, foot pointing forward wider than hip-distance width.
3. **Move arms to Cloud Hands Position:** raise right hand on inside, palm facing chest. Lower left hand on outside, palm facing belly.
   Then move to Wide Horse Stance, Center Position: shift weight evenly onto both feet. Rotate pelvis and trunk to center.
4. **Move to Wide Horse Stance with T'ai Chi Fold:** shift weight 100 percent onto right foot. Rotate pelvis and trunk to right diagonal.
   Simultaneously move arms into Holding the Ball Position: right hand chest height, palm facing down; left hand belly height. palm facing up.
5. **Move to Horse Stance with T'ai Chi Fold:** move left foot toward right; foot pointing forward.

6. **Move arms to Cloud Hands Position:** raise left hand on inside, palm facing chest; lower right hand on outside, palm facing belly.
   Then move to Horse Stance, Center Position: (see above).
7. **Move to Horse Stance with T'ai Chi Fold:** shift weight 100 percent onto left foot as pelvis and trunk rotate to left diagonal.
   Simultaneously move arms into Holding the Ball Position: left hand chest height, palm facing down; right hand belly height, palm facing up.

Corresponding Movement Pattern

- **Bear Rooting** (see page 24).
- **T'ai Chi Fold** (see page 30).
- **Holding Moon** (see page 34).

Modifications from Yang Style

- Side step is to the right instead of to the left, as in the traditional form.

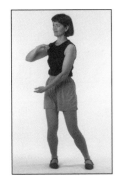 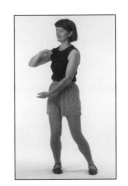 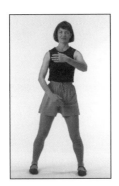 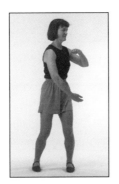 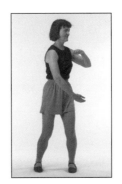 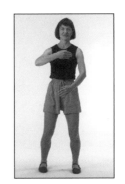 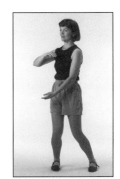

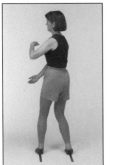 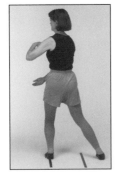 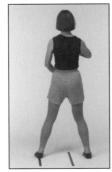 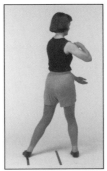 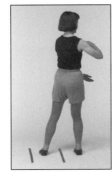 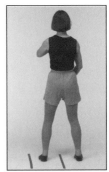 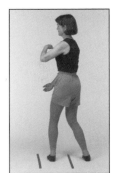

1. Horse Stance with T'ai Chi Fold; arms in Holding the Ball Position

2. Wide Horse Stance with T'ai Chi Fold

3. Wide Horse Stance, Forward Position; arms in Cloud Hands Position

4. Wide Horse Stance with T'ai Chi Fold; arms in Holding the Ball Position

5. Horse Stance with T'ai Chi Fold

6. Horse Stance, Forward Position; arms in Cloud Hands Position

7. Horse Stance with T'ai Chi Fold; arms in Holding the Ball Position

Single Whip

Movements

1. **Begin in Horse Stance with T'ai Chi Fold:** weight 100 percent on left foot; pelvis and trunk face left diagonal. **Arms in Holding the Ball Position:** left hand chest height, palm facing down; right hand belly height, palm facing up.

2. **Move to Closed Diagonal Position:** step forward with right foot pointing to left diagonal.

3. **Move to Closed Diagonal with T'ai Chi Fold:** shift weight 100 percent onto right foot. Rotate pelvis and trunk to right diagonal.
   Simultaneously move arms into Holding the Ball, Hook Position: right hand chest height, left hand belly height; fingers of right hand touch thumb.

4. **Transition:** rotate trunk and pelvis to neutral position, facing direction of right foot.
   Simultaneously extend Hook Hand: to the side, shoulder height.

5. **Move into 70/30 Stance, Back Position:** keeping 100 percent of the weight on the right foot, step with left foot, facing 90 degrees to the left of foot direction in **Cloud Hands.**

6. **Move into 70/30 Stance, Forward Position:** shift more weight (70 percent) onto left foot; rotate pelvis and trunk into neutral position, facing the direction of the left foot.
   Simultaneously move arms into Single Whip Position: raise left arm in front of body, then move fingers up. Turn palm to face forward, elbow bent in front of body, wrist neutral, palm facing forward and slightly down. Right arm remains in hook at right side.

Corresponding Movement Pattern

- **70/30 Stance** (see page 26).
- **T'ai Chi Fold** (see page 30).

Modifications from Yang Style

- The right foot steps forward to the left diagonal, eliminating the heel pivot.
- Right arm is positioned directly at right of body instead of at rear diagonal.

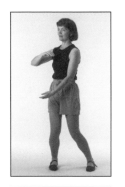 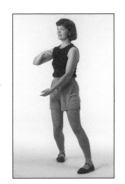 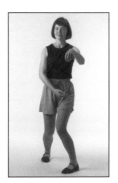 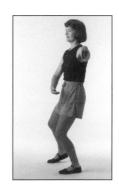 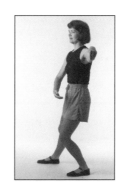 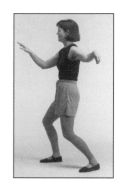

Front/Side View:
Mirror Image

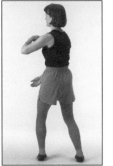 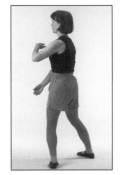 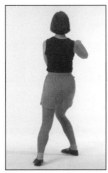 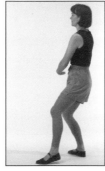 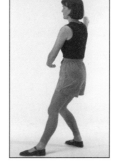 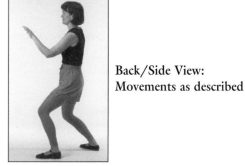

Back/Side View:
Movements as described

1. Horse Stance with T'ai Chi Fold; arms in Holding the Ball Position

2. Closed Diagonal Position

3. Closed Diagonal with T'ai Chi Fold; arms in Holding the Ball, Hook Position

4. Transition Position; arms extend in Hook Position

5. 70/30 Stance, Back Position

6. 70/30 Stance, Forward Position; arms in Single Whip Position

T'ai Chi Fundamentals Form: Section Three

Corresponding Movement Patterns:

All from Sections One and Two
Flying Crane
Softball Pitch
Dancing Crane

Snake Slides Down

Movements

1. **Begin in 70/30 Stance, Forward Position:** with more weight (70 percent) on left foot. Pelvis and trunk are in neutral position, facing the direction of the left foot. **Arms in Single Whip Position:** left palm faces forward, elbow bent in front of body, wrist neutral, palm facing forward and slightly down. Right arm at shoulder height, facing at the right side of the body. Right hand makes a hook with fingers touching thumb.

2. **Move to 70/30 Stance, Back Position with T'ai Chi Fold:** shift weight 100 percent onto right foot. Rotate pelvis and trunk to right diagonal. **Simultaneously move arms into Snake Slides Down Position:** left hand at inside of left thigh, palm facing right; right hand remains in a hook with fingers touching thumb.

Corresponding Movement Pattern

- **Softball Pitch** (see page 42).

Modifications from Yang Style

- Feet maintain the **70/30 Stance** during the weight shift to the back leg.
- The low squat position is eliminated.

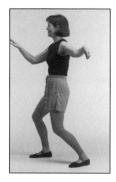

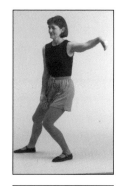

Side View:
Mirror Image

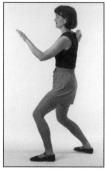

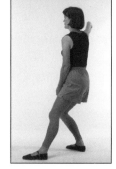

Side View:
Movements as described

1. 70/30 Stance,
Forward Position;
arms in Single
Whip Position

2. 70/30 Stance,
Back Position
with T'ai Chi
Fold; arms in
Snake Slides
Down Position

Golden Pheasant Stands on One Leg
(Left and Right Positions)

Movements

1. **Begin in 70/30 Stance, Back Position with T'ai Chi Fold:** pelvis and trunk face the right diagonal in the **T'ai Chi Fold.** Feet are in the **70/30 Stance** with 100 percent of the weight on the back foot.
   Arms in Snake Slides Down Position: left hand inside left thigh, palm facing right. Right arm at shoulder height, facing at the right side of the body. Right hand makes a hook with fingers touching thumb.

2. **Move to Open Diagonal Position:** rotate pelvis and trunk toward center as left heel pivots, pointing foot to left diagonal. Right knee maintains alignment over foot.

3. **Transition**: Shift weight 100 percent onto foot at left diagonal. Left knee maintains alignment over foot.
   Simultaneously move arms: move left arm forward as right arm drops to side.

4. **Move Into Flying Crane Position:** raise right knee in front of body, bringing foot off ground. Pelvis balanced, facing forward with shoulders aligned over hips. Right knee faces forward. The unweighted foot can touch the floor for balance if necessary.
   Simultaneously move arms into Golden Pheasant Position: raise right arm, elbow bent, palm facing left, fingers pointing up and forward. Left forearm and hand move parallel to left thigh.

5. **Transition:** step back to diagonal with right foot, toes first. Shift weight 100 percent onto right foot.

6. **Move Into Flying Crane Position:** raise left knee in front of body bringing foot off ground. Pelvis is balanced, facing forward with shoulders aligned over hips. Left knee faces forward. The unweighted foot can touch the floor for balance if necessary.
   Simultaneously move arms into Golden Pheasant Position: raise left arm, elbow bent, palm facing right, fingers pointing up and forward. Right forearm and hand move parallel to right thigh.

Corresponding Movement Pattern

- **Flying Crane** (see page 38).

Modifications from Yang Style

- Foot movements are simplified in transition from **Snake Slides Down.**
- The unweighted foot can touch the floor for balance.

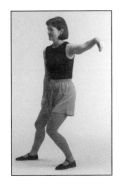
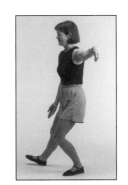
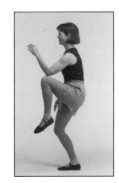
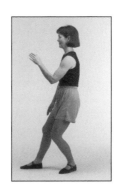
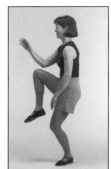

Side View:
Mirror Image

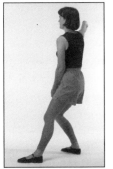
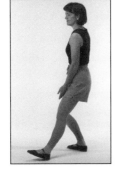
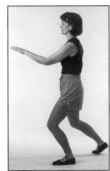
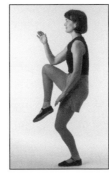
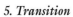
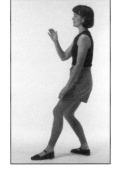

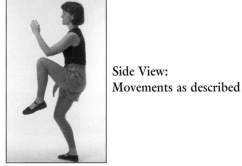

Side View:
Movements as described

1. 70/30 Stance,
Back Position
with T'ai Chi
Fold; arms in
Snake Slides
Down Position

2. Open Diagonal
Position

3. Transition

4. Flying Crane
Position; arms in
Golden Pheasant
Position

5. Transition

6. Flying Crane
Position; arms in
Golden Pheasant
Position

Separate Arms and Kick (Right and Left)

Movements

1. **Begin In Flying Crane Position:** right foot at diagonal, hips and shoulders facing forward; left knee is raised, facing forward.
   Arms in Golden Pheasant Position: left elbow bent in front of body, wrists neutral, palm facing forward and slightly down. Right forearm and hand parallel to right thigh.

2. **Transition:** step back to diagonal with left foot, toes first. Shift weight 100 percent onto left foot.
   Simultaneously cross wrists: palms facing to sides and down, chest height. Right arm on the outside, left arm on the inside.

3. **Move to Dancing Crane Position** (diagonal kick): lift right leg to right diagonal. Foot extends beyond the knee. Toes can touch the ground for balance if necessary.
   Simultaneously move arms into Separate Arms Position: left arm at side of body with elbow shoulder height. Right arm over right thigh with elbow at waist height. Palms face each other. Look to the right.

4. **Transition:** step back to diagonal with right foot, toes first. Shift weight 100 percent onto right foot.
   Simultaneously cross wrists, palms facing sides: cross wrists at chest height; left arm outside, right arm inside.

5. **Move to Dancing Crane Position** (diagonal kick): lift left leg to left diagonal. Foot extends beyond the knee. Toes can touch the ground for balance if necessary.
   Simultaneously move arms into Separate Arms Position: right arm at side of body with elbow shoulder height. Left arm over left thigh with elbow at waist height. Palms face each other. Look to the left.

Corresponding Movement Pattern

- **Dancing Crane** (see page 44).

Modifications from Yang Style

- Arm movements are simplified.
- The rotation of the trunk over the weighted leg is eliminated during the transitions before the kicks.

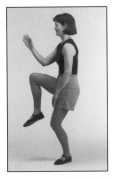
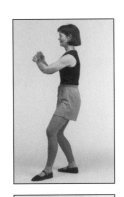
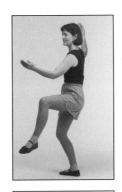
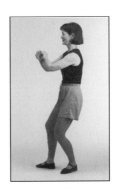
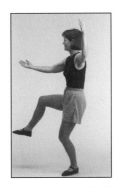

Side View:
Mirror Image

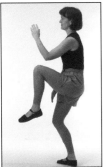
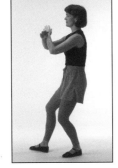
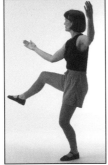
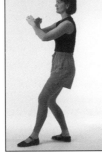
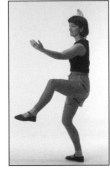

Side View:
Movements as described

*1. Flying Crane
Position; arms in
Golden Pheasant
Position*

*2. Transition
Position; wrists
crossed, palms fac-
ing sides*

*3. Dancing Crane
Position; arms in
Separate Arms
Position*

*4. Transition;
wrists crossed
palms facing sides*

*5. Dancing Crane
Position; arms in
Separate Arms
Position*

Brush Knee and Twist (Left)

Movements

1. **Begin in Dancing Crane Position** (diagonal kick): left knee faces left diagonal. Foot extends beyond the knee. Toes can touch the ground for balance if necessary.
   Arms in Separate Arms Position: right arm at side of body with elbow shoulder height. Left arm over left thigh with elbow at waist height. Palms face each other. Look to the left.

2. **Move to 70/30 Stance, Back Position with T'ai Chi Fold**: rotate pelvis and trunk to right diagonal. Step forward with left foot into **70/30 Stance, Back Position**, keeping weight 100 percent on right foot.
   Simultaneously move arms into Brush Knee Line-Up Position: bend right elbow so fingers point forward in the direction of the left foot. Circle left hand down in front of right thigh, palm faces left.

3. **Move to 70/30 Stance, Forward Position:** shift weight forward onto the left foot (70 percent) with the knees maintaining a flexed position. As weight shifts, the pelvis and trunk rotate to face forward in the direction of the left foot.
   Simultaneously move arms into Brush Knee, Push Position: move right arm forward lowering elbow to front of body, palm facing forward and down. Move left forearm and hand parallel to left thigh.

4. **Move to 70/30 Stance, Back Position with T'ai Chi Fold:** rotate pelvis and trunk to right diagonal, shifting weight 100 percent onto right foot.
   Simultaneously move arms into Brush Knee, Open Position: swing right arm to side, elbow shoulder height with palm facing forward. Move left hand in front of right hip, palm faces left.

5. **Move Arms into Brush Knee, Line-Up Position:** bend right elbow so fingers point forward in the direction of the left foot. Move left hand down in front of right thigh.

6. **Move to 70/30 Stance, Forward Position:** (see above).
   Simultaneously move arms into Brush Knee Push Position: (see above).

Corresponding Movement Pattern

- **70/30 Stance with Tai Chi Fold** (see page 40)
- **Softball Pitch** (see page 42).

Modifications from Yang Style

- The movements are repeated twice in succession.

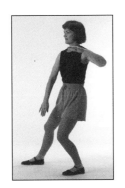
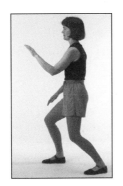
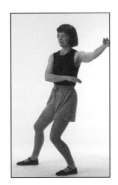
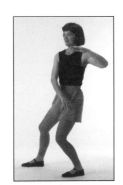
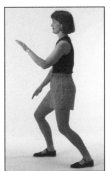
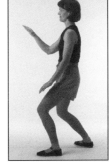

Side View:
Mirror Image

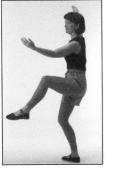
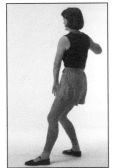
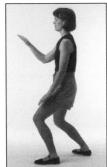
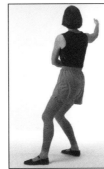
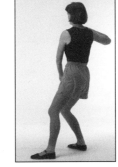
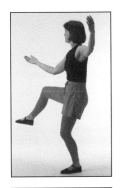

Side View:
Movements as described

1. Dancing Crane Position; arms in Separate Arms Position

2. 70/30 Stance, Back Position with T'ai Chi Fold; arms in Brush Knee, Line-Up Position

3. 70/30 Stance, Forward Position; arms in Brush Knee, Push Position

4. 70/30 Stance, Back Position with T'ai Chi Fold: arms in Brush Knee, Open Position

5. 70/30 Stance, Back Position with T'ai Chi Fold; arms in Brush Knee, Line-Up Position

6. 70/30 Stance, Foreward Position; arms in Brush Knee, Push Position

Brush Knee and Twist (Right)

After the transition, this movement is identical to the preceding movement except that it is done with the right foot forward.

Movements

1. **Begin in 70/30 Stance:** with more weight (70 percent) on the left foot.
   Arms in Brush Knee, Left Position: right arm forward with elbow bent, palm facing forward and down. Left forearm and hand are parallel to left thigh.

2. **Transition:** shift weight 100 percent onto right foot. Pivoting on left heel, turn trunk, pelvis and left foot to left diagonal. Right knee maintains alignment with foot.
   Simultaneously move arms into Brush Knee, Open Position: swing left arm to side, elbow shoulder height, palm facing forward. Circle right hand in front of left hip, palm facing to right.

3. **Move to 70/30 Stance, Back Position:** shift weight 100 percent onto left foot. Move right foot forward into **70/30 Stance** keeping weight 100 percent on left foot.
   Simultaneously move arms into Brush Knee, Line-Up Position: bend left elbow so fingers point forward in the direction of the right foot. Move right hand down in front of left thigh.

4. **Move into 70/30 Stance, Forward Position:** shift forward into **70/30 Stance** with more weight on right foot. As weight shifts, pelvis and trunk rotate to face forward in the direction of the right foot.
   Simultaneously move arms into Brush Knee, Push Position: move left arm forward lowering elbow to front of body, palm facing forward and down. Move right forearm and hand parallel to right thigh.

5. **Move to 70/30 Stance, Back Position with T'ai Chi Fold:** shift weight 100 percent onto left foot; rotate pelvis and trunk to left diagonal.
   Simultaneously move arms into Brush Knee, Open Position: (see above).

6. **Move arms into Brush Knee, Line-Up Position:** (see above).

7. **Move into 70/30 Stance, Forward Position:** (see above).
   Simultaneously move arms into Brush Knee, Push Position: (see above).

Corresponding Movement Pattern

- **70/30 Stance with Tai Chi Fold** (see page 40)
- **Softball Pitch** (see page 42).

Modifications from Yang Style

- The arm and trunk movements are repeated twice in succession.

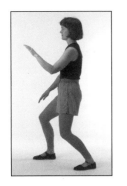
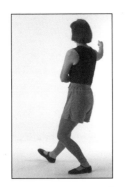
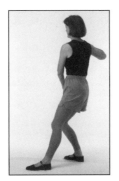
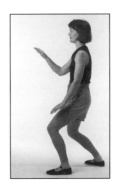
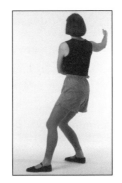
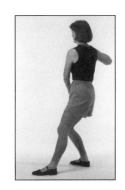
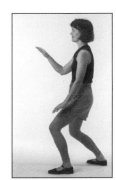

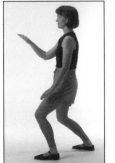
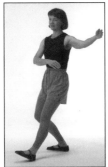
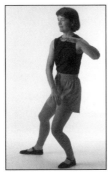
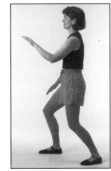
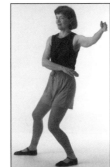
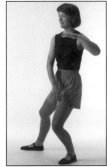
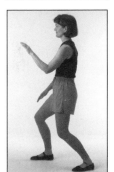

1. 70/30 Stance; arms in Brush Knee, Right Position

2. Transition; arms in Brush Knee, Open Position

3. 70/30 Stance, Back Position; arms in Brush Knee, Line-Up Position

4. 70/30 Stance, Forward Position; arms in Brush Knee, Push Position

5. 70/30 Stance, Back Position with T'ai Chi Fold; arms in Brush Knee, Open Position

6. 70/30 Stance, Back Position; arms in Brush Knee, Line-Up Position

7. 70/30 Stance, Forward Position; arms in Brush Knee, Push Position

Punch

Movements

1. **Begin in 70/30 Stance, Forward Position:** with more weight (70 percent) on right foot.
    Arms in Brush Knee, Push Position: left elbow bent in front of body, wrist neutral, palm facing forward and down; right forearm and hand parallel to right thigh.
2. **Transition:** shift weight 100 percent onto left foot. Pivoting on right heel, turn trunk, pelvis and foot to right diagonal. Left knee maintains alignment with left foot **Simultaneously move right hand into loose fist:** with fingers curled, thumb bent on outside. Left palm moves to face down and to right diagonal.
3. **Move to 70/30 Stance, Back Position with T'ai Chi Fold:** shift weight 100 percent onto right foot. Step with left foot forward into **70/30 Stance.**
4. **Move to 70/30 Stance, Forward Position:** shift weight forward onto the left foot (70 percent) with the knees maintaining a flexed position. As weight shifts, the pelvis and trunk rotate to face forward in the direction of the left foot.
    Simultaneously move arms into Punch Position: right hand moves forward into position at midline, forearm parallel to ground. Left elbow is bent with palm facing right forearm.

Corresponding Movement Patterns

*   70/30 Stance with Tai Chi Fold (see page 40)
*   Softball Pitch (see page 42).

Modifications from Yang Style

*   **Deflect Downward** and **Parry** movements are eliminated.

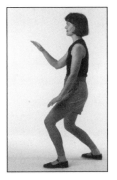 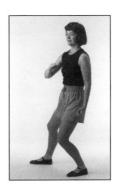 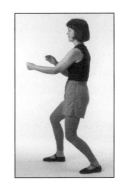 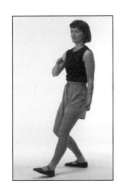

Side View:
Mirror Image

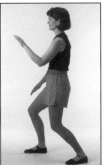 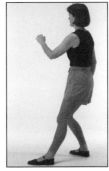 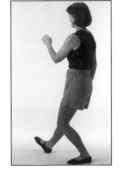 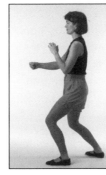

Side View:
Movements as described

*1. 70/30 Stance,
Forward Position;
arms in Brush
Knee, Push
Position*

*2. Transition;
right hand in fist*

*3. 70/30 Stance,
Back Position
with T'ai Chi
Fold*

*4. 70/30 Stance,
Forward Position;
arms in Punch
Position*

Withdraw and Push

Movements

1. **Begin in 70/30 Stance, Forward Position:** with more weight (70 percent) on the left foot.
   Arms in Punch Position: right fist faces forward at midline. Left elbow is bent with palm facing right forearm.

2. **Transition:** shift weight 50 percent onto right foot.
   Simultaneously move arms to cross horizontally: extend right arm, open palm. Move left wrist under right forearm, palm up.

3. **Move to 70/30 Stance, Back Position with T'ai Chi Fold:** shift weight 100 percent onto right foot; rotate pelvis and trunk to right diagonal.
   Simultaneously uncross hands horizontally: bend right elbow, draw right hand over left wrist.

4. **Move to 70/30 Stance, Back Position:** rotate trunk and pelvis to face the direction of the left foot.
   Simultaneously move arms to Push Position: parallel to each other, elbows heavy, wrists neutral, palms facing forward and slightly down.

5. **Move into 70/30 Stance, Forward Position** (see above).
   Arms remain in Push Position (see above).

Corresponding Movement Patterns

- *70/30 Stance with T'ai Chi Fold* (see page 40).

Modifications from Yang Style

- The weight shift and the turning of the trunk and pelvis are modified.
- Arm movements are modified.

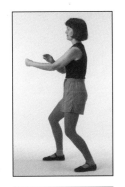
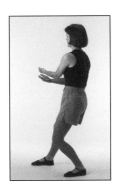
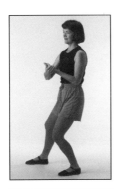
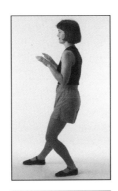
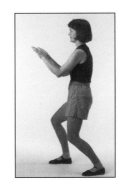

Side View:
Mirror Image

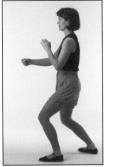
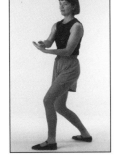
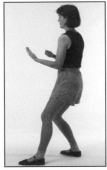
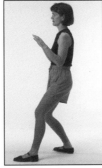
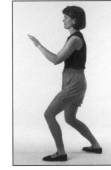

Side View:
Movements as described

1. 70/30 Stance, Forward Position; arms in Punch Position

2. Transition: arms cross horizontally

3. 70/30 Stance, Back Position with T'ai Chi Fold; arms uncross

4. 70/30 Stance, Back Position; arms in Push Position

5. 70/30 Stance, Forward Position; arms in Push Position

Cross Hands

Movements

1. **Begin in 70/30 Stance:** with more weight (70 percent) on left foot.
   Arms in Push Position: parallel to each other, elbows heavy, wrists neutral, palms facing forward and down

2. **Move to 70/30 Stance, Back Position:** shift weight 100 percent onto right foot.
   Simultaneously extend arms: extend elbows; palms face down, fingers face forward.

3. **Move to Closed Diagonal with T'ai Chi Fold:** keeping weight 100 percent on right foot, rotate pelvis and trunk 90 degrees to right, facing direction of the original starting position.
   Simultaneously raise arms: right arm moves to right side of body, left arm at left side of body. Both arms are raised, palms facing forward.

4. **Transition:** shift weight 100 percent onto left foot and pivot on right toes to face direction of left foot.
   Simultaneously circle arms: both arms circle out and down in front of body.

5. **Move to Horse Stance, Center Position:** move right foot back, hip-distance from left foot. Both feet point forward. Shift weight to center, evenly distributed over both feet, knees slightly bent.
   Simultaneously move arms to Cross Hands Position: as right root moves back, right arm moves under left. Both arms cross at midline, chest height. Palms face chest.

Corresponding Movement Patterns

- **70/30 Stance with Tai Chi Fold** (see page 40).
- **Horse Stance** (see **Posture**, page 14).

Modifications from Yang Style

- **None**

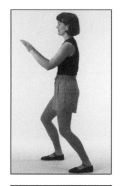
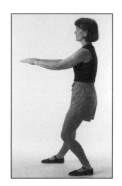
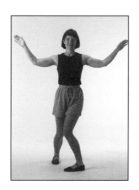
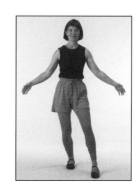
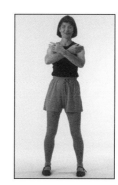

Side/Front View:
Mirror Image

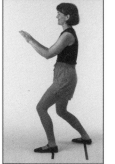
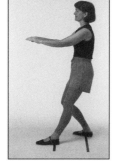
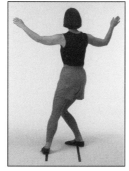
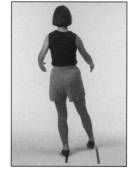
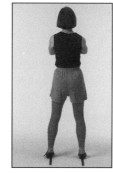

Side/Back View:
Movements as described

*1. 70/30 Stance,
Forward Position;
arms in Push
Position*

*2. 70/30 Stance,
Back Position;
arms straighten*

*3. Closed Diagonal,
T'ai Chi Fold
Position; arms raised*

*4. Transition; arms
circle*

*5. Horse Stance;
arms in Cross
Hands Position*

Closing Move

Movements

1. **Begin in Horse Stance, Center Position:** weight evenly
   distributed on both feet with knees slightly bent.
   Arms in Cross Hands Position: wrists cross at midline;
   palms facing chest.
2. **Straighten knees slightly.**
   Simultaneously move arms into Energetic Position: at
   sides, elbows slightly bent, fingers pointing down and forward.
3. **Move to Open and Stable Position:** bend knees and
   shift weight 100 percent onto left leg. Pivot on right heel,
   pointing foot to right diagonal. Left knee maintains alignment with left foot.
4. **Move into 'V' Position:** shift weight 100 percent onto
   right foot. Move left foot into diagonal position next to
   right foot so that the heels touch. Shift weight to center
   and straighten knees slightly.
5. **End with feet in 'V' position:** body upright and relaxed
   with heels together at a 45 degree angle; weight evenly
   distributed on both feet.
   Arms relaxed: hanging at sides.

Corresponding Movement Patterns

- **Horse Stance** (see **Posture,** page 14).
- **Open and Stable Move** (see page 22).

Modifications from Yang Style

- **None**

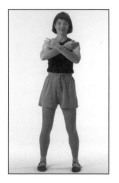
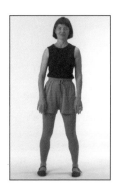
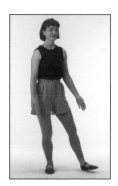
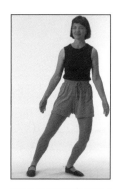
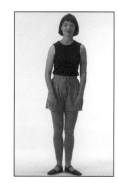

Front View:
Mirror Image

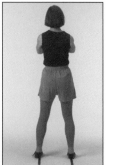
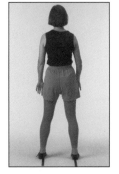
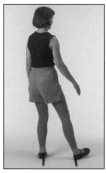
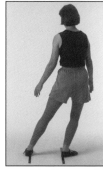
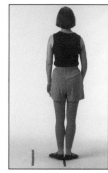

Back View:
Movements as described

1. Horse Stance; arms in Cross Hands Position

2. Arms in Energetic Position

3. Open and Stable Position

4. Feet in "V" Position, single weighted

5. Feet in "V" Position; arms relaxed at sides

CHAPTER FOUR

The Mind/Body Principles of T'ai Chi

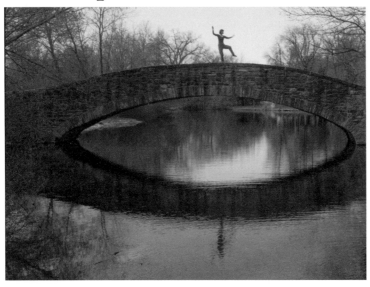

Description

This chapter includes suggestions for daily practice and explores elements of T'ai Chi that apply to physical and mental function as well as relationship to community and environment.

T'ai Chi is based on the perspective that mind and body are not separate; rather, they are different expressions of *Qi* energy or life force. In addition, the cosmos, the earth and all forms of life on earth are also different expressions of the same life force. According to the principles of T'ai Chi, all life is interconnected. The principles that facilitate health of body naturally are healthy for the mind, and visa versa. These principles apply to human interaction as well. T'ai Chi was developed as a means of cultivating the body, mind and spirit to function in harmony with the external world.

Names of Principles

Section One:
Active Relaxation

Centering
Relaxed Alertness
Stillness within Movement

Reminders for T'ai Chi Practice

Section Two:
Effective Action

Body Mechanics
Spontaneous Action
Moving around Obstacles

Section Three:
Energetics

Heavy and the Light
Relaxed and Rooted
The String of Pearls

Mind/Body Principles Section One: Active Relaxation

Centering

T'ai Chi is practiced beginning with a few moments of quiet with focus on slow, natural breathing to help calm the mind, relax the body and bring attention fully into the present moment. The practitioner notes subtle changes within the body while tuning the senses to the external environment. This process is an essential component of all T'ai Chi practice recommended at the beginning and end of each teaching session. It is also an important part of individual daily practice routines.

Ideally, T'ai Chi is practiced in silence or with quiet, calming background music. Watching television, listening to programs on headphones or playing loud music is counterproductive to this process. It distracts us from what we are doing. It disconnects the mind from the body. Taking time to focus our attention is best done without external distractions.

This simple **Centering** process helps develop increased mental focus. It facilitates mind/body integration, reinforces natural diaphragmatic breathing patterns and enhances postural alignment. It can be practiced at any time, taking as little as a few seconds, or it can be practiced as a three-to-five-minute standing *Qigong* meditation. It is an effective stress-reduction technique, and a means of heightening sensory awareness and assessing our emotional responses.

To review essential elements of **Centering**, see Chapter Two: **Posture** (page 14) and **Breathing** (page 16).

Centering

Attention to the present moment

Breath awareness

Relaxation

Body upright and naturally aligned

Awareness of hands and feet

Bring your attention into the present moment. Feel the movement in your body as you breathe. The belly relaxes, the breath sinks. Let your head feel suspended from above. Keeping your body upright, sink your weight into the balls and heels of your feet. Feel into the palms and fingers of your hands. Now, lets begin.

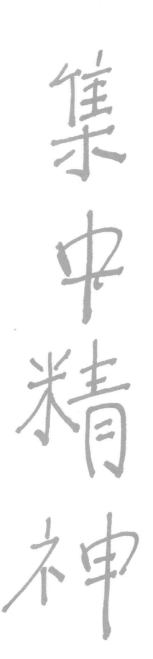

Relaxed Alertness

T'ai Chi trains the practitioner to relax in the midst of activity. Although it is based in martial arts blocks, kicks and punches, T'ai Chi is done deliberately and slowly, with a peaceful, quiet mind.

T'ai Chi is practice of relaxed alertness in motion. Being relaxed is often associated with being unfocused or sleepy. However, when we are focused in the present and disengaged from concerns of the past and anxiety about the future, we are relaxed and alive to each moment. We are awake, aware and responsive to what is occurring in any given moment.

When we are alert, relaxed and alive to the present moment, we function optimally. We can feel a greater sense of vitality and connection to our environment and to others. According to Chinese medical theory, these conditions increase our experience of energy or *Qi*. We can feel the *Qi* flowing. We experience ourselves as being "in the flow" of life.

Relaxed Alertness

Quiet

Alert

As we practice each section, we can reflect on the inner process of T'ai Chi.
The mind rests peaceful in quiet; alert and calm while in motion.

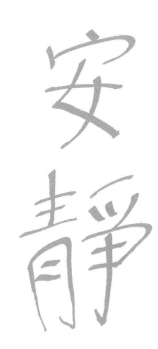

Stillness Within Movement

The mountain and the river are two powerful images that express the essence of staying both relaxed and alert in the midst of activity. Training the mind and body to be quiet is a characteristic discipline in Asian martial arts and meditation. It is a skill that takes practice and is developed over time. It is an essential ingredient for developing clear intention and follow-through, and for staying on track with our goals and purpose. Cultivating stillness can contribute to healthy emotional balance and effective decision-making skills. When we practice being quiet, we are less likely to be influenced by impulsive personal whim or by distractions in the external environment.

According to the philosophy of the *Tao,* when we are still both mentally and physically, we create minimal disturbance in the external environment. We have greater access to our intuitive and intellectual resources and can assess any situation before acting.

Our resulting actions may be appropriate, effective and powerful. Our movements flow naturally, without resistance, in an uninhibited and harmonious manner. They arise not from need or desire, but from inner peace.

Stillness Within Movement

Be still as a mountain.

Move like a great river.

T'ai Chi combines relaxed fluid motion with inner tranquillity.
The spirit is strong, resilient and internally gathered.
The movement flows naturally.

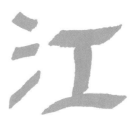
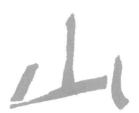

Mind/Body Principles Section Two: Effective Action

Body Mechanics

T'ai Chi strengthens the body with minimal stress to the joints. Its principles and movements actually retrain our natural alignment, and reinforce proper body mechanics inherent in virtually all activity.

This is a description of all natural, effective movement. Developing "root" involves both mental and physical integration. Physical balance and stability are enhanced both by proper physical alignment and by maintaining awareness of the feet. The power of the movement comes from the legs which have the largest muscles in the body. The head, trunk and pelvis stay upright and relaxed, reducing stress on the back, hips and shoulders. The movement of the arms and hands is largely determined by the turning of the trunk and pelvis.

Often we think of strong arms as the source of physical power. However, the arms are as relaxed as possible, serving as a conduit for the action.

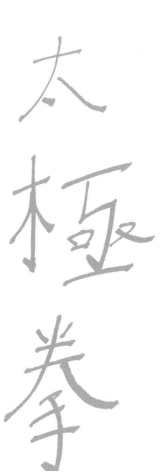

Body Mechanics

The motion is
Rooted in the feet
Powered by the legs
Directed by the torso
Expressed in the hands

The soles of the feet are the root; the firm and stable legs release and trigger the motion.
With the lower back relaxed, the trunk and pelvis rotate like a wheel, directing the
action into the arms, hands and fingers. The feet, legs and torso act simultaneously so
that the timing and position are naturally coordinated.

Spontaneous Action

This is a "top-down" perspective of T'ai Chi movement that emphasizes the importance of feeling the uplift at the crown. The head, trunk and pelvis are the vertical column. When this column is both upright, "as if suspended from above," and well rooted, we naturally initiate movement from the vertical central axis. With the body relaxed and aligned, spontaneous movements are naturally circular.

"Intention is aligned and firm" indicates that we keep life in perspective. According to the philosophy of the *Tao*, or way of nature, our actions are most effective and appropriate when we include the Three Treasures of Life in our ongoing awareness. They are "Heaven, Earth and Human." "Heaven" is our personal source of spiritual strength, the vastness of space, or the knowledge that we are all One. "Earth" is our collective home, which gives birth to and supports many forms of life. As humans standing between Heaven and Earth, we function best when remembering that these Three Treasures are an integral part of every moment of life.

This is the principle of aligned intention and firm balance. Spontaneous actions that reflect awareness of Heaven, Earth and other Humans are likely to "follow the circle," or be a response that is harmonious for both the immediate circumstance and for the broader context, or circle of life.

Spontaneous Action

Aligned and firm
Be Spontaneous
Circular

The head and trunk are like a vertical column rotating from its central axis. When intention is aligned and firm, spontaneous action naturally follows the circle.

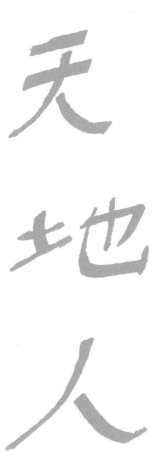

Moving Around Obstacles

When the mind is quiet, the energy or *Qi* is gathered and focused. We are fully present, alive to whatever is occurring at the moment. We often resist whatever is occurring and wish that it were some other way. This can dissipate our energy, or disperse our *Qi*. It inevitably results in being less in touch with our situation.

When we accept the reality that is occurring at any given moment, we experience a clearer perception of the situation that enables us to act appropriately. Attempting to force a fixed, preconceived plan often leads to further depletion of our energy, and doesn't necessarily bring results. We can move through obstacles more easily when we accept what is happening and move with, rather than against, the reality of the moment.

Water is the element in nature that expresses this. Water takes the form of any vessel: yielding, flowing, resisting nothing. Yet it moves with tremendous power as a waterfall, or as ocean waves in a storm. Water resists nothing. It goes with the flow. When we detach from our need to control outcomes according to our fixed plans, we become more fluid, receptive and clear. We have an unlimited range of responses to what is occurring.

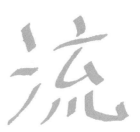

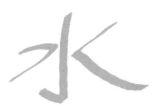

Moving Around Obstacles

Seek stillness
Move with the flow

Seek the peaceful stillness beneath all thought and desire.
Study water as it flows freely around all obstacles: fluid motion, inner tranquillity.

Mind/Body Principles Section Three: T'ai Chi Energetics

The Heavy and the Light

Like the **Centering** exercise in Section One, the "Three Heavies" and "Three Lights" reinforce integration of body and mind and helps cue key elements for relaxation and for the flow of *Qi*. In addition, they promote increased sensory awareness and may contribute to better physical balance.

When any part of the body is relaxed, it feels heavier. The lower back is relaxed so the tailbone is heavy and enhances stability. Knees are soft, slightly bent, shoulders relaxed, elbows heavy. Keeping the elbows relaxed and heavy helps keep the shoulders relaxed and facilitates the flow of *Qi* into the hands and fingers. Maintaining a feeling of heaviness in the coccyx and knees helps develop "root." Developing "root" involves relaxation, physical stability and an energetic sense of connection to the earth. This is called *Sung* in Chinese.

"Light" can be interpreted to mean both "bright" and "not heavy." The uplift at the crown is a universal cue for spiritual awareness. The sense of uplift at the crown also enhances posture and balance. Keeping the eyes light reminds us to maintain awareness of the external environment while focusing internally.

Qi is most easily felt in the hands. When the hands are "bright and filled with energy," they may feel heavy, pulsing, tingling, warm or as if there is an increased sense of touch or a sense of magnetic attraction or repulsion between them. These are indications that we are experiencing sensory awareness of our *Qi* energy flowing.

The Heavy and the Light

The Three Lights:
Crown — Eyes — Fingers

The Three Heavies:
Tailbone — Knees — Elbows

Let the crown of your head feel light and uplifted, your eyes awake and bright, your hands and fingers alive and filled with energy. Relax your lower back so your tailbone feels heavy and rooted to the earth. Knees are soft and slightly bent, shoulders are relaxed, elbows heavy.

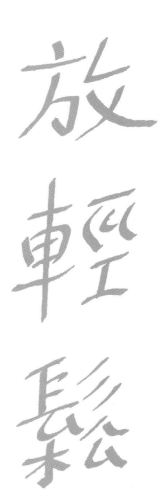

Flexible and Rooted

The use of imagery can be helpful in experiencing a sense of stability and expansiveness. The tree is an ideal metaphor for our bodies and may be useful when practicing T'ai Chi: our legs are the trunk with roots extending deep into the earth. These roots draw nutrients into the trunk and out into the branches. What is firmly rooted is easy to nourish. Our branches reach up to absorb the light of the sun. We are nurtured by the earth and the light of the sun. Relaxed and rooted, our branches sway effortlessly in the breeze.

The trunk and pelvis are aligned, moving effortlessly while resting on firm and stable legs. The legs and feet do the work. When the upper body feels relaxed and aligned, the weight sinks directly into the legs and feet. This helps maintain balance with minimal stress to the joints. When the upper body is tense, it is more difficult to sense this natural alignment. When they are relaxed and "floating," the trunk and pelvis simply go along for the ride.

Flexible and Rooted

Relaxed

Rooted

Like a floating cloud

Relaxed and rooted to the earth, the body moves like a floating cloud,
or like a tree branch blowing in the breeze.

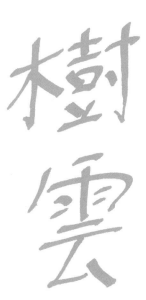

The String of Pearls

This describes some of the energetics for optimum flow of *Qi*. Pearls are a symbol for longevity and immortality in China. The bones are the pearls, the joints are the thread. The muscles and tendons are relaxed, moving with minimal effort. The slow movement gently cleanses the synovial fluid that lubricates the joints. In Chinese medicine, the *Qi* of the joints can become stagnant or blocked by inactivity and by tension. Moving with loose and relaxed joints promotes the flow of *Qi*, enhancing health and well-being.

Mental states also influence the flow of *Qi* in the body, in relationships and the environment. All life is interconnected like a string of pearls.

The String Of Pearls

Loose

Lively

The breathing is deep and long. The bones and joints are connected like a string of pearls: light, nimble and loosely strung together. With this effortless motion, relaxed and lively, there is space for the energy to flow.

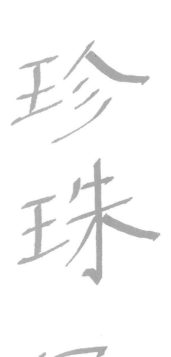

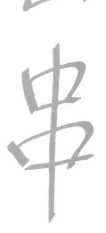

Reminders for T'ai Chi Practice

T'ai Chi is an ideal exercise for lifelong well-being. Daily practice is the key to reaping its many benefits. When we regard T'ai Chi as a form of personal hygiene, like brushing our teeth and combing our hair, we get into the habit of routine practice. We can do it almost anywhere, at any time. It takes no special equipment and very little time.

Regular practice of T'ai Chi can create an oasis of calm in our lives. It provides us with time each day to nurture body and mind, and to reflect on the gift of life. Each practice session, even if it is only two or three minutes, is most beneficial if it includes the following:

- Begin with a few moments of **Centering** (see page 100).
- During practice, relax and move slowly.
  If there is less time, do fewer movements.
  It is counterproductive to speed them up!!
- After practice, take a few more moments for quiet or contemplate any of the Mind/Body Principles discussed in this chapter.

May we all become strong as the oak, flexible as the willow and clear as still water.

Reminders for T'ai Chi Practice

Practice every day

Feel the flow

Check for accuracy

Remember principles and perspectives

To reap the benefits of T'ai Chi, do it everyday. A regular time and place that supports your practice can help you maintain the habit. Spend as much time feeling the flow of the movements as you do checking for accuracy of the form. During your T'ai Chi practice, or at any time, choose a principle or perspective to focus on. It can apply to all activities and life situations .

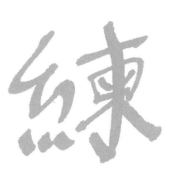
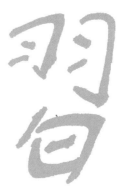

Appendix

Glossary Of Chinese Terms

Bai Hui : Hundred Channels Point
The Crown point at the top of the head.

Dan Tien (also spelled *Tan T'ien*): Vital Energy Field
Literally "Cinnabar Field." *Dan* means Cinnabar or deep red, *Tien* is field. Also known as Elixir Field.
In T'ai Chi, reference to the *Dan Tien* usually refers to the *Lower Dan Tien* However, the body has three:
> The *Lower Dan Tien* is in the belly. It is the personal energy field.
> The *Middle Dan Tien* is in the chest. It is the interpersonal energy field.
> The *Upper Dan Tien* is in the head. It is the spiritual energy field.

Kwa (also spelled *Gua*): the hip joint
The place where the hip joint forms a crease at the top of the femoral triangle. It is a key area of focus in T'ai Chi.

Laogong (also spelled *Lao Kung*): Labor Temple
Point in center of palm for expressing energy through the hands. It is an acupuncture point. It also corresponds to the sweet spot for hands-on healing.

Qi (also spelled *Ch'i* or *Chi*): Vital Energy or Life Force
It is the energy that permeates all living things. It is a commonly used term in everyday Chinese language.
For example:
> Weather: *tien qi* or heaven energy; Air: *kung qi* or empty energy; Air conditioner: *lung qi ji* or cold energy machine; Angry: *sheng qi* or energy rising.

Qigong (also spelled *Ch'i Kung*): Vital Energy Cultivation
This term is used for a wide a variety of moving, standing or sitting exercises for promoting the flow of *Qi* in the body. T'ai Chi is a form of *Qigong*.

Sung: Active Relaxation
This term also means to sink. It is a state of being both calm, alert and energetic.

T'ai Chi (also spelled *Taiji*) : Supreme Ultimate
The unifying still point, the Grand Terminus or Ridge Post connecting the heavens and earth.

T'ai Chi Ch'uan (also spelled *Taijiquan*): Supreme Ultimate Boxing
T'ai Chi means: the unifying still point, the Grand Terminus or Ridge Post connecting the heavens and earth. *Ch'uan* or *Quan* means boxing or fist.

Tao (also spelled *Dao*): Way or Path. The ancient Chinese philosophy of the Middle Way. The natural path for harmony and longevity.

Yong Quan (also spelled *Yung Ch'uan*): Bubbling Well
Root or balance point energetically connecting to the earth *Qi*. It is located in the middle of the sole of the foot, one-third anterior and two-thirds posterior, when the foot is in plantar flexion. It is also an acupuncture point.

Summary of Research on T'ai Chi Ch'uan

Current research indicates that practice of T'ai Chi can improve balance, reduce falls and increase leg strength. In addition it can enhance cardiovascular, respiratory and immune function and promotes emotional well-being. It also has been found to lower blood pressure and cortisol levels.

Cardiovascular

- Low-to-moderate-intensity exercise. *(Zho 1982)*
- Safe exercise for individuals at high risk for cardiovascular disease. *(Schneider 1991)*
- May delay decline of cardiorespiratory function in older adults. *(Lai 1995)*
- May be prescribed as suitable aerobic exercise for older adults. *(Lai 1993)*
- Most recommended aerobic exercise for coronary artery disease. *(Ng 1992)*
- Significant reduction in both systolic and diastolic blood pressure. *(Channer 1996)*

Respiratory

- Enhanced ventilary capacity without cardiovascular stress. *(Brown et al 1995)*
- Efficient use of ventilatory volume, efficient breathing patterns. *(Schneider 1991)*

Stress Hormones (Salivary Cortisol Levels)

- Significant drop during and after practice. *(Jin 1989, 1992)*

Immune Response (Blood T-Cells)

- Marked increase during and after practice. *(Sun 1989)*

Mood States (Self-Reports)

- Reduced tension, anxiety, fatigue, depression and confusion. *(Jin 1989)*
- Improved mood states, reduction of anxiety states. *(Jin 1992)*

Balance

- Improved strength, mobility, balance, endurance. *(Tse 1992)*
- Significant improvement in balance maintained. *(Wolfson 1996)*

Reduced Falls

- Reduced falls by 47 percent. reduced fear of falling. *(Wolf 1996)*

Weight-Bearing Exercise

- No exacerbation in joint symptoms of individuals with rheumatoid arthritis. *(Kirstens 1991)*
- Alternative exercise therapy as part of rehabilitation program. *(Kirstens 1991)*

Research References

Brown DD, Mucci WG, Hetzler RK, Knowlton RG. Cardiovascular and ventilatory responses during formalized T'ai Chi Ch'uan exercise. *Research Quarterly for Exercise & Sport.* 1989;60:246-250.

Brown DR, Wang Y, Ward A, et al. Chronic effects of exercise and exercise plus cognitive strategies. *Med Science Sports Exercise* 1995;27:765-775.

Channer KS, Barrow D, Barrow R, Osborne M, Ives G. Changes in hemodynamic parameters following T'ai Chi Chuan and aerobic exercise in patients recovering from acute myocardial infarction. *Postgraduate Medical Journal* . 1996;72:349-351.
Gong LS et al. Changes in heart rate and electrocardiogram during taijiquan exercise. *Chinese Medical Journal.* 1981;94(9): 589-592.

Jin P. Changes in heart rate, noradrenaline, cortisol and mood during T'ai Chi. *Journal of Psychosomatic Research.* 1989;33:197-206.

Jin P. Efficacy of t'ai-chi, brisk walking, meditation, and reading in reducing mental and emotional stress. *Journal of Psychosomatic Research.* 1992;36:361-370.

Judge JO, Lindsey C, Underwood M, Winsemius D. Balance improvements in older women: effects of exercise training. *Physical Therapy.* 1993;73:254-262.

Kirsteins AE, Dietz F, Hwang SM. Evaluating the safety and potential use of a weight-bearing exercise, tai-chi chuan, for rheumatoid arthritis patients. *American Journal of Physical*

Medicine and Rehabilitation. 1991;70(3):136-141.
Kutner NG, Barnhart H, Wolf SL, McNeely, Xu T. Self-report benefits of tai chi practice by older adults. *Journal of Gerontology.* 1997;52(5): 242-46.

Lai JS, Wong MK, Lan C, Chong CK, Lien IN. Cardiorespiratory responses of t'ai chi chaun practitioners and sedentary subjects during cycle ergometry. *Journal of Formosan Medical Association.* 1993;92:894-899.

Lai JS, Lan C, Wong MK, Teng SH. Two-year trends in cardiorespiratory function among older t'ai-chi chuan practitioners and sedentary subjects. *Journal of American Geriatric Society.* 1995;43:1222-1227.

Lan C, Lai JS, Chen SY, Wong MK. Twelve-month tai chi training in the elderly: its effects on health and fitness. *Medicine & Science in Sports & Exercise.* 1998;30(3): 345-51.

Ng RK. Cardiopulmonary exercise: a recently discovered secret of t'ai chi. *Hawaii Medical Journal.* 1992;51:216-217.

Province MA, Hadley EC, Hornbrook MC, et al. The effects of exercise on falls in elderly patients. A preplanned meta-analysis of the FICSIT Trials. Frailty and injuries: cooperative Studies of Intervention Techniques. *Journal of the American Medical Association.* 1995;273:1341-1347.

Ross MC, Preswalla JL. The therapeutic effects of tai chi for the elderly. *Journal of Gerontological Nursing.* 1998;24(2):45-7.

Schneider D, Leung R. Metabolic and cardiorespiratory responses to the performance of wing chun and t'ai-chi chuan exercise. *International Journal of Sports Medicine.* 1991;12(3):319-23.

Sun XS, Xu Y, Xia YJ. Determination of E-rosette-forming lymphocytes in aged subjects with Taichiquan exercise. *Intenational Journal of Sports Medicine* .1989;10:217-219.

Tse S, Bailey DM. T'ai Chi and postural control in the well elderly. *Am Journal of Occupational Therapy*. 1992;46:295-300.

Wolf SL, Kutner NG, Green RC, McNeely E. The Atlanta FICSIT study: two exercise interventions to reduce frailty in elders. *Journal of the American Geriatric Society*. 1993;41:329-332.

Wolf SL, Barnhart HX, Kutner NG, McNeely E, Coogler C, Xu T. Reducing frailty and falls in older persons: an investigation of T'ai Chi and computerized balance training. *Journal of the American Geriatric Society*. 1996;44:599-600.

Wolfson L, Whipple R, Judge J, Amerman P, Derby C, King M. Training balance and strength in the elderly to improve function. *Journal of the American Geriatric Society*. 1993;41:341-343.

Wolfson L, Whipple R, Derby C, Judge J, King M, Amerman P, Schmidt J, Smyers D. Balance and strength training in older adults: intervention gains and T'ai Chi maintenance. *Journal of the American Geriatric Society*. 1996;44:498-506.

Zhou DH. Preventive geriatrics: an overview from traditional Chinese medicine. *American Journal of Chinese Medicine*. 1982;10:32-39.

Zhou D, Shephard RJ, Plyley Mj, Davis GM. Cardiorespiratory and metabolic responses during Tai Chi Chuan exercise. *Canadian Journal of Applied Sport Sciences*. 1984;9:7-10.

References for Quotes from T'ai Chi Masters and Mind/Body Principles

Chen, William. *Body Mechanics of T'ai-Chi Ch'uan*. Wm. CC Chen, 2 Washington Square Village #10J, New York 10012; Eighth edition 1999.

Jou,Tsung Hwa. *The Tao of T'ai-Chi Ch'uan*. Warwich NY: T'ai-Chi Foundation;1988.

Lo, Benjamin et al. (Trans.) *The Essence of T'ai-Chi Ch'uan*. Berkeley: North Atlantic Books;1985.

Mitchell, Stephen, (Trans.)*Tao Te Ching*. New York: Harper and Rowe;1988.

Ueshiba, Morihei. *The Art of Peace*. John Stevens. (Trans) Boston: Shambala;1992.

Recommended Reading

Books

Bottomley, Jennifer. T'ai-Chi: Choreography of Body and Mind, in *Complementary Therapies in Rehabilitation: Holistic Approaches for Prevention and Wellness*. (C. Davis ed.) Thorofare, New York: Slack Inc.;1997.

Cheng, Man-Ching and Smith, Robert. *T'ai-Chi*. Rutland, Vermont: Tuttle;1967.

Delza, Sophia, T'ai Chi Ch'uan, in *Illustrated Encyclopedia of Body-Mind Disciplines*. (N. Allison ed.) New York: Rosen Publishing; 1999.

Kline, Bob. *Movements of Magic*. Newcastle Publishing Co;1984.

Liang, T.T. *T'ai-Chi Ch'uan for Health and Self-Defense*. Boston: Redwing;1974.

Lo, Benjamin and Inn, Martin. (Translators) *Cheng Tzu's Thirteen Treaties on T'ai-Chi Ch'uan*. Berkeley: North Atlantic Books;1985.

Lowenthal, Wolfe. *Gateway to the Miraculous*. Berkeley: North Atlantic Books;1988.

Lowenthal, Wolfe. There *Are No Secrets: Professor Cheng Man Ch'ing and His T'ai-Chi Ch'uan*. Berkeley: North Atlantic Books;1991.

Wile, Douglas. *Master Cheng's Thirteen Chapters on T'ai-Chi Ch'uan*. Brooklyn: Sweet Chi Press;1982.

Articles

Tai Chi. *Harvard Women's Health Watch*. 1996; Nov: 4.

Balance Exercises: Staying Steady on Your Feet. *Mayo Clinic Health Letter*. 1998; Feb:4-5.

Davis, Meryl. Cool Moves. *Remedy*. 1997; May-June:18-21.

Downs, Linda. T'ai-Chi. *Modern Maturity*. 1992; June-July:61-64.

LePostolle, Mark. Complimentary Movement Therapies. *Advance for Physical Therapists 1998;* August 17: 8-10.

Ramsay, Susan Morrill. T'ai-Chi as a Balance Tool, Part One. *Advance for Physical Therapists*. 1998; August: 5, 35.

Ramsay, Susan Morrill. T'ai-Chi as a Balance Tool, Part Two. *Advance for Physical Therapists*. 1998; September 7.

Rizzo, Angelo. Before the Fractures. *PT Magazine*. 1996; May:128.

Sarola, Tony. Taijiquan and Western Physiological Thought, *Qi: The Journal of Traditional Eastern Health and Fitness*. 1991; Summer: 8-10.

Scott, Abigail. Improving Motion and Emotion. *Advance for Speech-Language Pathologists and Audiologists*. 1998; February:15,16,23.

Shine, Jerry. T'ai-Chi: A Kinder, Gentler Workout. *Arthritis Today*. 1993; Jan-Feb:31-33.

Swartzman, Leonard. T'ai-Chi and Parkinson's Disease. *Parkinson's Report*. 1996; Vol XVII 1st quarter: 22-23.

Thompson, LaDora. Current Literature Reviews: Did you Even Think that T'ai-Chi Could be used as a Therapeutic Intervention? *Gerinotes* . 1996:V3 no 4: 26.

Woodworth, Barbara. T'ai-Chi-Possibilities for Occupational Therapy. *Occupational Therapy Forum*. 1990; Vol Vno. 40: 1-4.

About the Authors

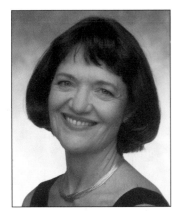

Tricia Yu, MA, creator of the **T'ai Chi Fundamentals Program**, is director of the T'ai Chi Center in Madison, Wisconsin, one of the oldest and largest schools in the United States. Teaching T'Chi, Qigong and meditation has been her primary occupation for the past 28 years. Tricia received her Bachelor of Arts degree in psychology from DePauw University in Indiana, and her Master of Arts in education from Claremont Graduate School in California. In 1970 she began her study of T'ai Chi and meditation with Taoist Master Liu Pei Chung. Since returning to the United States her teachers include Yang Style T'ai Chi masters Benjamin Pang Jeng Lo and William C.C. Chen; she is certified by Master Chen. Tricia is co-author of the **ROM Dance Range of Motion Exercise and Relaxation Program** which integrates elementary T'ai Chi principles into a medical model therapeutic exercise and pain management program. She has also produced two videos for the general public: **T'ai Chi: Exercise for Lifelong Health and Well-Being**, and **Energize: Daily Warm-ups for Flexibility and Strength**. She presents trainings on these programs nationally.

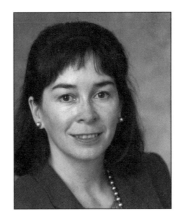

Jill Johnson, MS, PT, GCS, is a geriatric clinical specialist in physical therapy at the New England Center for Integrative Health. She received both her Bachelors of Science in physical therapy and Masters in biomechanics from the University of Wisconsin-Madison. Jill has published numerous research articles on geriatric rehabilitation and has received a grant from the Physical Therapy Foundation to study falls in the elderly. She teaches both yoga and T'ai Chi and uses them in her professional practice. She was instrumental in adapting the ROM Dance into versions for seated and supine use and presents ROM Dance and T'ai Chi Fundamentals training workshops nationally.

Resources by Tricia Yu

T'ai Chi and Warm-Up Instructional Materials

These represent a body of work from 28 years experience teaching T'ai Chi. They were produced in 1999.

T'ai Chi Fundamentals: for Health Care Professionals and Instructors

This video and instructional manual translate the Fundamentals Form and the Movement Patterns of the above video for instructors who will teach these exercises to patients and students. Jill Johnson, a physical therapist, analyzes the movements, their clinical applications, and functional benefits using Western medical terminology. The instructional manual provides detailed form instruction, expands discussion on therapeutic applications, mind/body principles, and describes modifications from traditional Yang Style T'ai Chi.

T'ai Chi Fundamentals: Simplified Exercises for Beginners

This video teaches the basic Movement Patterns inherent in traditional T'ai Chi, and offers step-by-step instruction in the Fundamentals Form. Tricia adapted these routines from the Yang Style Form, creating a systematic approach for mastering T'ai Chi basics. It is suitable for a wide range of abilities and experience.

T'ai Chi: Exercise for Lifelong Health and Well-Being

This video reviews the traditional Yang Style Short Form, its principles and philosophy in beautiful settings and in a clear and easy-to-learn format. It is designed to complement class instruction and is a useful resource for all levels of experience.

Energize: Daily Warm-Ups for Flexibility and Strength

This video provides instruction and guided practice in short routines that Tricia practices every day. The exercises range from simple stretches to more advanced exercises for T'ai Chi practitioners.

The ROM Dance Materials

In 1981 Tricia collaborated with Diane Harlowe, MS, OTR, FAOTA, an occupational therapist to create the **ROM Dance Range of Motion and Pain Management Program.** It is a medical model therapeutic exercise program that is used in hospitals, clinical settings, geriatric facillities and home health. It is designed for people with fibromyalgia, arthritis, lupus and other painful or limiting conditions. The following ROM Dance instructional materials integrate elementary principles of T'ai Chi, imagery, and music into this innovative exercise program.

ROM Dance Illustrated Text

The ROM Dance: A Range of Motion Exercise and Relaxation Program by Diane Harlowe and Tricia Yu, 1984, 1992, 1997. 120 pp.

ROM Dance Instructional Video Tapes

The following video tapes, created in 1994, begin with a performance of the ROM Dance and then offer step-by-step instruction for home or group practice.

The ROM Dance in Sunlight is the original version of the ROM Dance with images of sunlight, warm water, and friendship.

The ROM Dance in Moonlight is an adaptation for people with Lupus or sun sensitivity, and includes images of moonlight, water, and friendship.

The ROM Dance: Seated Version is an adaptation for wheelchair use. It also includes **The ROM Dance in Sunlight** for patients who will progress to a standing position. Additionally, it offers suggestions for further adaptations by physicians and therapists.

The ROM Dance: An Overview (1984) includes segments of a ROM Dance health education class for older adults with rheumatoid arthritis. It is designed to stimulate interest in participation.

ROM Dance CDs and Audio Tapes

The following audio tapes integrate healing imagery and sensory awareness in guided relaxation exercises. They are also for personal or group practice of the ROM Dance once the basic movements have been learned.
ROM Dance in Sunlight Body Awareness and Breathing
ROM Dance in Moonlight Soothing Meditation
ROM Dance Seated Version Body Awareness and Breathing

Music CDs and Audio Tapes

These background music tapes are composed and performed by Tricia Yu.
Reflections is calming and uplifting.
Waves and Gentle Currents is peaceful and relaxing.

For further information, contact:
Uncharted Country Publishing 1-800-488-4940
P.O. Box 3332, Madison, Wisconsin 53704-0332

Visit our web sites at:
ROM Dance: www. romdance.com
T'ai Chi Center: www.taichihealth.com